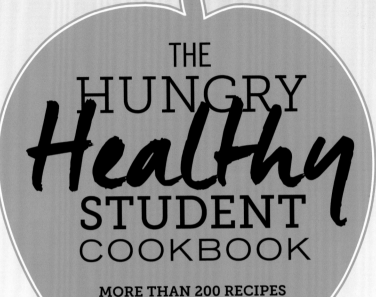

THE HUNGRY *Healthy* STUDENT COOKBOOK

MORE THAN 200 RECIPES THAT ARE DELICIOUS AND GOOD FOR YOU TOO

spruce

An Hachette UK Company
www.hachette.co.uk

First published in Great Britain in 2016 by Spruce,
an imprint of Octopus Publishing Group Ltd
Carmelite House
50 Victoria Embankment
London EC4Y 0DZ
www.octopusbooks.co.uk

ISBN 978-1-84601-513-7

A CIP catalogue record for this book is available from the British Library

Printed and bound in China

10 9 8 7 6 5

The recipes in this book have been labelled as suitable for Gluten Free,
Vegan and Vegetarian diets. Vegetarians should look for the 'V' symbol on
a cheese to ensure it is made with vegetarian rennet. There are vegetarian
forms of Parmesan, Feta, Cheddar, Cheshire, Red Leicester, dolcelatte and
many goats' cheeses, among others.

Standard level spoon measurement are used in all recipes.
1 tablespoon = one 15 ml spoon
1 teaspoon = one 5 ml spoon

Both imperial and metric measurements
have been given in all recipes. Use one
set of measurements only and not a mixture
of both.

Ovens should be preheated to the specific
temperature – if using a fan-assisted oven,
follow manufacturer's instructions for
adjusting the time and the temperature.

Pepper should be freshly ground black
pepper unless otherwise stated.

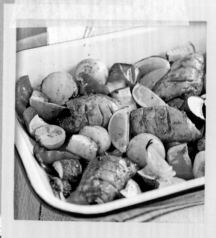

SPICED ROAST CHICKEN WITH LIME

Contents

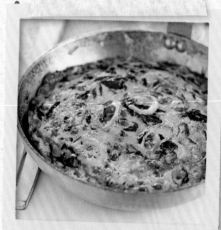

SPINACH & PEA FRITATTA

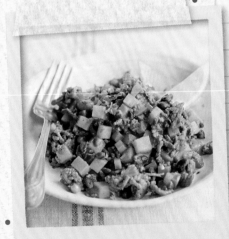

WEST INDIAN BEEF & BEAN STEW

INTRODUCTION

Leaving home and living on your own for the first time is both challenging and exciting. And while you're settling in, meeting new people and getting to grips with your independence, food can swiftly slide down the list of priorities. But it's important to establish good habits from the beginning and try to incorporate healthy eating as part of a healthy lifestyle. It's no more expensive or time consuming to eat healthily as a student; it just takes a bit more planning. So, if you want to enjoy a varied diet that doesn't have to be emptied on to your plate from a polystyrene tub, it's time to up your game in the kitchen and get to grips with ingredients and cooking techniques.

COOKING FOR YOURSELF

Whether you live on campus or in shared accommodation, you'll need to be organized when it comes to budgeting and shopping for food. If you're moving in with people you already know then it makes sense to work out what kitchen equipment you'll need and divide the list between you. That way, you won't end up with six juicers and an empty crockery cupboard. Likewise, when it comes to shopping, your budget will stretch much further if you pool your resources and shop as a household. You can buy ingredients in bulk and make the most of buy-one-get-one-free deals. However, you will need to take individual preferences and diets into account – it's hardly fair if the vegetarian among you has to fund a weekly meat feast.

FOODIE FRICTION

Food can be the cause of tension in shared student houses so it's a good idea to set out a few simple rules when you first move in. That doesn't mean installing CCTV in the fridge and keeping your favourite cereal in a safe in case anyone tries

to tuck into a bowl for breakfast. But it does mean working out a cooking and shopping rota, if you're going to eat meals together. You'll need to decide on a feasible weekly food budget and allocate someone to take control of it. You obviously won't all be eating at home every night of the week so you could, for example, club together for midweek meals and then let everyone fend for themselves at the weekend.

WHERE TO SHOP

The internet makes it easy for a shared household to do their food shop. You can pick a time when everyone is around so you all get to have a say in what makes it into the trolley. A meal planner will make it much easier to shop to budget and if this is agreed in advance, there'll be fewer 'discussions' about which ingredients you need to buy. Shopping online means you don't all have to trek to the supermarket together – a particular drag if no one has a car. You can order your shopping in one go and get it delivered when you know someone will be at home.

Local markets and farmers' markets often offer value for money, especially for seasonal produce. This is a great way to shop for a special weekend meal, or local ingredients that you won't see in the supermarket.

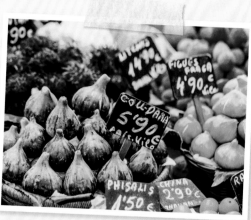

STOCK UP YOUR STORECUPBOARD

Your first grocery shop will probably be the most expensive, as you'll need to stock up on storecupbo ard essentials that form the basis of many meals. Alternatively, as with equipment, you could devise a list and ask everyone to bring a few items when you move in. Here's the lowdown on what you should line your cupboards with on moving-in day.

- **CONDIMENTS** Salt and pepper are essential for many recipes and good seasoning will liven up most dishes. You will also need vegetable oil for cooking and olive oil for dressings and sauces. Ketchup, mayonnaise and mustard are also staples.

- **BUTTER** Toast is a student staple so a good supply of butter or margarine is essential. This is also an important ingredient for mash.

- **SPICES** You don't need a full range of spices in a student kitchen but if you stock up on chilli powder, turmeric, cumin and maybe some mustard and fennel seeds, you'll be able to rustle up a half decent curry. Stock cubes and bouillon powders are also handy when you don't have any fresh stock made up (see Back to Basics, pages 242–51).

- **ONIONS AND GARLIC** Like salt and pepper, onion and garlic are vital ingredients in all manner of dishes across all cuisines. These have a long shelf life if you keep them in the fridge.

- **PASTA AND RICE** Bakes, salads, risottos, curries, soups, pilafs... the list is endless and a good stock of pasta and rice will see you through the lean times.

- **PULSES AND GRAINS** Split peas, lentils, couscous, bulgar wheat and quinoa are fantastic storecupboard staples for meals in their own right, or used to bulk up soups and stews.

- **CANS** Cans of beans (kidney beans, butter beans, and so on), sweetcorn and chickpeas are dependable favourites when the budget is suffering. They are cheap and nutritious and can be swiftly turned into a curry or chilli with a few additional ingredients.

- **FREEZER STAPLES** A lot of student accommodation suffers from the lack of a decent freezer and you might have to make do with a couple of shelves or a small compartment at the top of the fridge. But as long as there's space for some frozen vegetables and a few tubs of leftovers you should be able to get by.

HEALTHY WEEK MEAL PLANNER

	MONDAY	TUESDAY	WEDNESDAY	THURSDAY	FRIDAY	SATURDAY	SUNDAY
BREAKFAST	MANGO & ORANGE SMOOTHIE (page 12)	BERRY, HONEY & YOGURT POTS (page 16)	MIXED GRAIN PORRIDGE (page 21)	MAPLE-GLAZED GRANOLA WITH FRUIT (page 20)	APPLE & YOGURT MUESLI (page 19)	CORN & BACON MUFFINS (page 26)	BANANA & SULTANA DROP SCONES (page 24)
LUNCH	TURKEY & AVOCADO SALAD (page 165)	FALAFEL PITTA POCKETS (page 37)	HEARTY MINESTRONE (page 48)	TANDOORI CHICKEN SALAD (page 164)	TUNA & SWEETCORN WRAPS (page 43)	BAKED SWEET POTATOES (page 84)	SPINACH & PEA FRITTATA (page 206)
DINNER	PASTA WITH SPICY LENTILS (page 129)	STEAMED GINGER FISH (page 198)	SMOKED MACKEREL SUPERFOOD SALAD (page 158)	RANCH-STYLE EGGS (page 70)	FAST CHICKEN CURRY (page 190)	FIVE VEGGIE PIZZA (page 211)	SWEDISH MEATBALLS (page 100)

ESSENTIAL EQUIPMENT

If you're starting from scratch you'll probably have to beg or borrow most of your kitchen equipment, which means you won't be cooking with state-of-the-art pans and processors. But you don't actually need many gadgets and gizmos to rustle up any of the recipes in this book. With just a few basics you can eat well and even impress your friends with more daring creations when you develop some culinary confidence. Here's a list of the equipment you'll need in order to avoid a bread and baked beans diet.

UTENSILS Measuring jug, two different-sized mixing bowls, wooden spoon, rolling pin, grater, spatula, chopping board, vegetable peeler, whisk, colander, sharp knives (one small for prepping veg and one large for chopping, slicing bread etc).

POTS AND PANS Large and small saucepan (with lids), large nonstick frying pan, steamer (very useful but a metal colander over a pan will work fine). A wok is also handy for quick stir-fries, but not essential.

COOKWARE Baking sheet, roasting tin, flameproof casserole dish, large rectangular ovenproof dish (for lasagnes, bakes etc), wire cooling rack, cake tins, muffin tin and pastry cutters (if you're a baker).

A blender or food processor is a luxury item that will prove useful if you find your cooking mojo. But don't worry if you can't get your hands on these pricier pieces of culinary kit – a relatively inexpensive hand blender will do the job for most soups and smoothies and your knife skills will be all the better for chopping everything by hand.

FIVE A DAY

It's common knowledge that we should all aim to eat at least five portions of fresh fruit and vegetables every day but it's easy to lose track, particularly when you're busy working and socializing, and grabbing food on the go. However, if you want to stay healthy, this is a quick and easy way to cram plenty of vitamins and minerals into your diet.

HIGH FIVE

1 Get in the habit of having fruit with breakfast and you've already earned one of your five before you leave the house - this could be chopped fruit on muesli or granola, a glass of fresh juice, or a banana on your cornflakes or porridge.

2 Steam vegetables as an accompaniment to dinner or have a side salad.

3 Switch your usual mid-morning bag of crisps for some chopped carrots and hummus.

4 Try ordering a fruit smoothie instead of that double-shot latte – you'll get the same buzz while upping your daily dose of fruit.

5 Tuck into a baked potato or toast piled high with baked beans - pulses count as one portion so there's no need to miss out on a lunchtime fave.

HEALTHY HABITS

It's easy to get into bad habits when you're responsible for all your own food shopping and meal prep. You might have the best intentions about staying healthy and eating a nutritious and balanced diet, but when you're dashing straight from the lecture theatre to the pub, or you're craving a sugar hit to get you through a marathon essay-writing session, it's easy to fall off the wellbeing wagon and reach for salty snacks, energy drinks and chocolate bars.

SUGAR RUSH Sugar offers a short-term solution to lethargy but it won't keep you company for very long, as the initial buzz is swiftly followed by an energy lapse and a craving for more sugary junk food. It's the added sugars in food and drink that are the real enemy, especially if the food doesn't have any other redeeming nutritional features. Food labelling is becoming more transparent, so always check the label to see just how much sugar the product contains and to give yourself a reality check and a nudge to choose a healthier alternative.

Fizzy drinks, processed snacks, some breakfast cereals and pasta sauces are all major culprits, but making simple changes like switching to porridge for breakfast, making your own sauce and cutting out the unnecessary biscuits and chocolate bars can all make a big difference. And do you really need two or three spoons of sugar in your morning coffee? Think of added sugar as empty calories – something your body doesn't need and something you can easily train it not to crave.

CALL TIME ON DRINKING A healthy lifestyle doesn't mean you have to treat your body like a temple 24/7. It's all about balance and making sensible choices most of the time. As long as you're aware of what you should be eating and drinking, the odd splurge or treat isn't the end of the world.

The same is true for drinking – student life wouldn't quite be the same if you sipped on a sparkling water in the union bar or slurped on smoothies at partiesand club nights. But it's important to know your limitations and be aware of the number of units you're drinking. They can quickly add up, even during the more innocuous evenings in the pub. So, if you're out a few times a week, you're likely to be drinking far more than the recommended government guidelines, which are 2-3 units per day for women and 3-4 units per day for men.

BUDGETING

Boring as it may be, unless you want to spend the last month of each term hiding in your hovel and eating plain rice, budgeting is a necessary part of student life. Each recipe in this book is rated from 1 to 3, with 1s providing end-of-term saviours that can be scraped together for a pittance, and 3s to splash out and impress all your friends.

Know your units

WOMEN (2-3 units) a day

1 pint average strength (4%) beer or cider

Medium (175ml) glass of wine

2-3 shots (25ml) of spirits

MEN (3-4 units) a day

1½ pints average strength (4%) beer or cider

Large (250ml) glass of wine

3-4 shots (25ml) of spirits

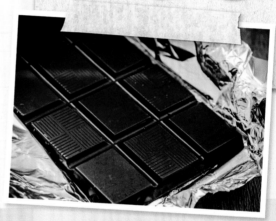

MOOD BOOSTERS

Leaving home for the first time is a major life event and while it signals a huge leap in your independence, it can also have a big impact on your emotional state. It's normal to feel homesick and, as previously mentioned, it's important to take care of yourself by eating well, exercising and not overindulging on the alcohol front. As you settle into your course you'll also be putting a lot of pressure on your brain, which makes it even more important to boost your body with bundles of vitamin-rich foods. If you're having a bad day, feeling tired and finding it difficult to concentrate, there are a few foods that can help lift you up and give you a boost. Here are five to get you started:

WATER We should drink about 1½-2 litres of fluid a day and the more of that amount that's made up of water, the better. A small drop in the amount of fluid you drink can very quickly affect your mood and you'll begin to get dehydrated, have a headache and feel tired.

DARK CHOCOLATE Yes, it does contain sugar, but dark chocolate also releases endorphins (happy chemicals) in your brain. Of course, everything in moderation so stick to a couple of squares – just enough to put a smile on your face.

OILY FISH Salmon, sardines, mackerel and tuna all contain omega-3, which is an important nutrient that can help enhance your mood by calming you down if you feel stressed.

GREEN TEA This should be your hot beverage of choice when you're revising for exams – the thiamine in green tea can help you concentrate.

CARBOHYDRATES These are a vital part of a balanced diet and if you cut out the carbs you might not feel on top form. Carbs help your brain to produce serotonin and a regular intake of slow-release, wholegrain carbohydrates will help to keep you focused and full of energy.

Brekky & Lunchbox

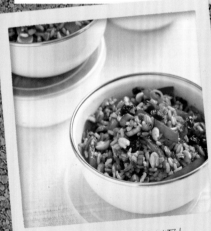

BROWN RICE SALAD WITH
PEANUTS & RAISINS

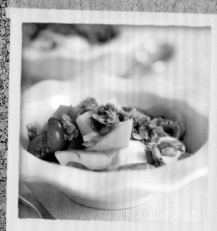

MAPLE-GLAZED GRANOLA WITH FRUIT

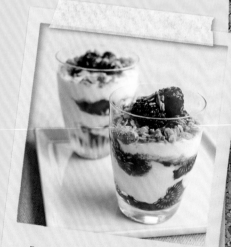

BERRY, HONEY & YOGURT POTS

BREAKFAST SMOOTHIE Ⓥ

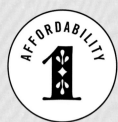
1 Place all the ingredients in a blender or food processor and blend until smooth and creamy.

2 Pour into 2-3 glasses and serve immediately.

1 tablespoon pomegranate juice
1 small ripe banana, peeled and sliced
300 ml (½ pint) soya milk
1 tablespoon almonds
1 tablespoon rolled oats
½ teaspoon clear honey
1½ teaspoons ground linseeds
2 tablespoons natural yogurt

Serves **2-3**
Prep time **10 minutes**

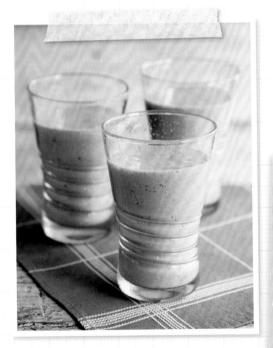

HEALTHY TIP
WAKE UP AND REHYDRATE Keep a large glass of water by your bed and drink it as soon as you wake up in the morning. This will help your body to rehydrate while you're getting ready for the day.

Banana & Peanut Butter SMOOTHIE

PEANUT BUTTER MAY SOUND AN UNUSUAL INGREDIENT IN A SMOOTHIE, BUT IN FACT IT COMBINES WONDERFULLY WELL WITH BANANAS TO MAKE A RICH, SATISFYING DRINK. PEANUTS CONTAIN RESVERATROL, PLANT STEROLS AND OTHER PHYTOCHEMICALS, WHICH, ACCORDING TO RESEARCH, HAVE CARDIO-PROTECTIVE AND CANCER-INHIBITING PROPERTIES. THIS HIGH-CALCIUM DRINK IS A GREAT PICK-ME-UP AFTER EXERCISE.

1 ripe banana
300 ml (½ pint) semi-skimmed milk
1 tablespoon smooth peanut butter or 2 teaspoons tahini

Serves **2**
Prep time **10 minutes, plus freezing**

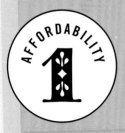

1 Peel and slice the banana, put it in a freezer-proof container and freeze for at least 2 hours or overnight.

2 Put the frozen banana, the milk and peanut butter or tahini in a blender or food processor and blend until smooth.

3 Pour into 2 glasses and serve immediately.

NUTRITIONAL TIP
Tahini is a delicious paste made from crushed sesame seeds. Weight for weight, sesame seeds contain ten times more calcium than milk. This smoothie is an excellent source of vitamins C, B1, B2, B6 and B12, folic acid, niacin, calcium, copper, potassium, zinc, magnesium and phosphorus.

MANGO & ORANGE SMOOTHIE

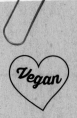

Vegan

1 ripe mango, peeled, stoned and chopped, or 150 g (5 oz) frozen mango chunks
150 ml (¼ pint) natural soya yogurt
150 ml (¼ pint) orange juice
finely grated rind and juice of 1 lime
2 teaspoons agave nectar, or to taste

Serves **2**
Prep time **10 minutes**

1 Blend together the mango, yogurt, orange juice, lime rind and juice and agave nectar in a blender or food processor until smooth.

2 Pour into 2 glasses and serve immediately.

VARIATION

For a ginger banana smoothie, blend together 1 ripe, peeled banana, 1.5 cm (¾ inch) piece of fresh root ginger, peeled and grated, 150 ml (¼ pint) natural soya yogurt and 150 ml (¼ pint) orange or mango juice in a blender or food processor until smooth. Sweeten to taste with agave nectar, pour into 2 glasses and serve immediately.

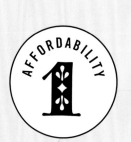

AFFORDABILITY
1

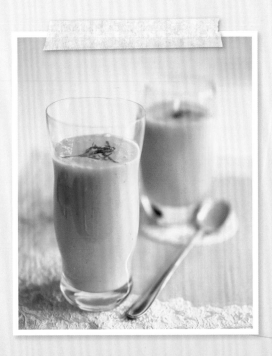

AVOCADO & BANANA SMOOTHIE Ⓥ

1 small ripe avocado
1 small ripe banana
250 ml (8 fl oz) skimmed milk

Serves **1**
Prep time **10 minutes**

1 Peel the avocado, remove the stone and roughly chop the flesh. Peel and slice the banana.

2 Place the avocado, banana and milk in a blender or food processor and blend together until smooth.

3 Pour into a glass, add a couple of ice cubes and serve immediately.

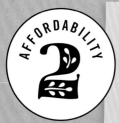

AFFORDABILITY 2

HEALTHY TIP

IN THE TROPICS, avocados are often called poor man's butter because of their creamy texture and high fat content. Unlike butter, though, most of the fat is monounsaturated – the sort that helps lower levels of the 'bad' cholesterol (or low-density lipoproteins) while raising levels of the 'good' cholesterol (or high-density lipoproteins). Just one avocado provides around half the recommended daily intake of vitamin B6. This smoothie is an excellent source of vitamins C, E, B1, B2, B6 and B12, as well as folic acid, calcium, potassium, copper, zinc, magnesium and phosphorus.

GINGERED APPLE & CARROT JUICE

Vegan

375 g (12 oz) carrots, peeled and cut into chunks

3 dessert apples, cored and cut into chunks

2.5 cm (1 inch) piece of fresh root ginger, peeled

Serves **2**
Prep time **10 minutes**

1   Feed the carrot and apple chunks through a juicer with the ginger.

2   Pour the juice into 2 glasses and serve immediately.

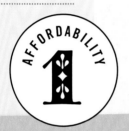

AFFORDABILITY **1**

HEALTHY TIP

THIS VIBRANT JUICE is packed with carotenoids. These are converted to vitamin A by the body. They are particularly important for normal tissue growth and are an antioxidant.

Watermelon Cooler

Vegan

100 g (3½ oz) watermelon

100 g (3½ oz) strawberries

100 ml (3½ fl oz) water

small handful of mint or tarragon leaves, plus extra to serve (optional)

Serves **2**
Prep time **10 minutes, plus freezing**

1   Skin and deseed the watermelon and chop the flesh into cubes. Hull the strawberries. Freeze the melon and strawberries until solid.

2   Put the frozen melon and strawberries in a blender or food processor, add the water and mint or tarragon and blend until smooth.

3   Pour the mixture into 2 glasses, decorate with mint or tarragon leaves, if liked, and serve immediately.

VARIATION
For a melon and almond smoothie, blend 100 g (3½ oz) frozen galia melon flesh with 100 ml (3½ fl oz) chilled, sweetened almond milk.

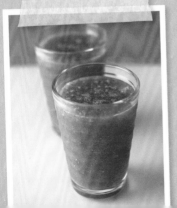

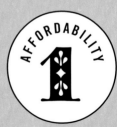

AFFORDABILITY **1**

Cucumber LASSI (V)

150 g (5 oz) cucumber
150 ml (¼ pint) natural yogurt
100 ml (3½ fl oz) ice-cold water
handful of mint
½ teaspoon ground cumin
squeeze of lemon juice

Serves **1**
Prep time **10 minutes**

1 Peel and roughly chop the cucumber. Place in a blender or food processor with the yogurt and iced water.

2 Pull the mint leaves off their stalks, reserving a few for decoration. Chop the remainder roughly and put them into the blender. Add the cumin and lemon juice and blend briefly until smooth.

3 Pour the smoothie into a glass, decorate with mint leaves, if liked, and serve immediately.

VARIATION
For mango lassi, cut the flesh of 1 ripe mango into cubes and add it to a blender or food processor with 150 ml (¼ pint) natural yogurt and the same amount of ice-cold water, 1 tablespoon rosewater and ¼ teaspoon ground cardamom. Blend briefly, then serve immediately.

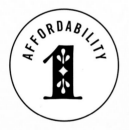

AFFORDABILITY

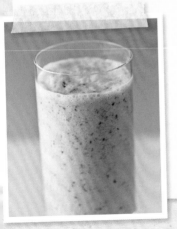

HEALTHY TIP
SMOOTHIE DOES IT If your fruit bowl is looking a little sad, with a couple of lonely items fast approaching over-ripeness, wash, peel, dice and slice and blitz them up into a liquid vitamin boost. Add a dash of orange juice or other fruit juice if you need to boost the volume.

BERRY, HONEY & YOGURT POTS ⓥ

1 Whizz half of the berries with the orange juice and honey in a blender or food processor until fairly smooth.

2 Transfer to a bowl and stir in the remaining berries.

3 Divide one-third of the berry mixture between 4 glasses or small bowls. Top with half of the yogurt.

4 Layer with half of the remaining berry mixture and top with the remaining yogurt.

5 Top with the remaining berry mixture, then sprinkle over the granola just before serving.

400 g (13 oz) frozen mixed
   berries, defrosted
juice of 1 orange
6 tablespoons clear honey
400 ml (14 fl oz) vanilla yogurt
50 g (2 oz) granola

Serves **4**
Prep time **10 minutes**

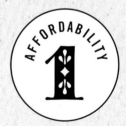

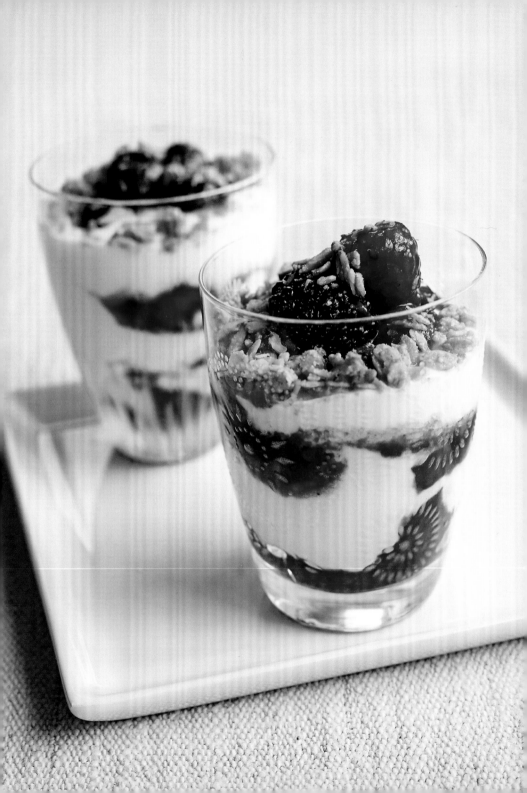

Blueberry, Oat & Honey
CRUMBLE Ⓥ

1 Put the butter in a 200 ml (7 fl oz) microwave-proof mug and microwave on full power for 30 seconds or until melted.

2 Stir in the oats, sugar, honey and cinnamon and microwave on full power for 1 minute.

3 Mix well, then stir in the blueberries and microwave on full power for a further 1 minute until the blueberry juices start to run. Serve with Greek yogurt.

1 tablespoon unsalted butter
50 g (2 oz) rolled oats
1 tablespoon soft light brown sugar
2 teaspoons clear honey
generous pinch of ground cinnamon
50 g (2 oz) blueberries
0%-fat Greek yogurt, to serve

Serves **1**
Prep time **2 minutes**
Cooking time **2½ minutes**

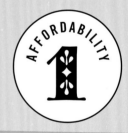

AFFORDABILITY 1

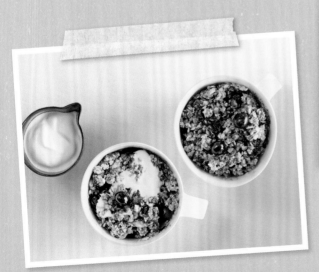

APPLE & YOGURT MUESLI 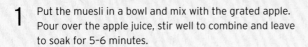 Ⓥ

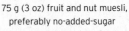

AFFORDABILITY
2

1 Put the muesli in a bowl and mix with the grated apple. Pour over the apple juice, stir well to combine and leave to soak for 5–6 minutes.

2 Divide the soaked muesli between 2 serving bowls and spoon the yogurt on top.

3 Scatter over the linseeds, if using, and serve with a drizzle of honey, if liked.

75 g (3 oz) fruit and nut muesli, preferably no-added-sugar
1 dessert apple, such as Granny Smith, peeled, cored and coarsely grated
200 ml (7 fl oz) chilled apple juice
125 ml (4 fl oz) 0%-fat Greek yogurt with honey

To serve
linseeds (optional)
clear honey (optional)

Serves **2**
Prep time **10 minutes, plus soaking**

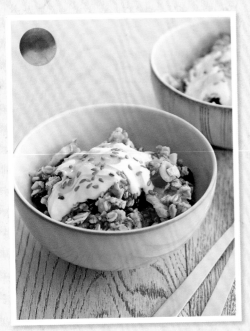

HEALTHY TIP

BULK UP BREAKFAST If you eat a hearty meal before heading into college you're less likely to crave unhealthy snacks during the morning. Think big — porridge, granola or muesli with some chopped fruit and natural yogurt should see you through until lunchtime.

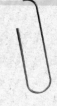

MAPLE-GLAZED
GRANOLA
WITH FRUIT

2 tablespoons olive oil
2 tablespoons maple syrup
40 g (1 ½ oz) flaked almonds
40 g (1 ½ oz) pine nuts
25 g (1 oz) sunflower seeds
25 g (1 oz) porridge oats
375 ml (13 fl oz) natural yogurt

Fruit salad
1 ripe mango, peeled, stoned and
  sliced
2 kiwifruit, peeled and sliced
small bunch of red seedless
  grapes, halved
finely grated rind and juice of 1
  lime

Serves **6**
Prep time **20 minutes, plus
cooling**
Cooking time **5-8 minutes**

1 Heat the oil in an ovenproof frying pan, then add the maple syrup, nuts, seeds and oats and toss together.

2 Transfer the pan to a preheated oven, 180°C (350°F), Gas Mark 4, and cook for 5-8 minutes, stirring once and moving the brown edges to the centre, until the granola mixture is evenly toasted.

3 Leave the mixture to cool, then pack it into a storage jar, seal, label and consume within 10 days.

4 Make the fruit salad. Mix the fruits with the lime rind and juice, spoon the mixture into bowls and top with spoonfuls of natural yogurt and granola.

AFFORDABILITY
2

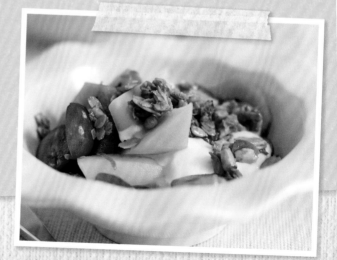

MIXED GRAIN
PORRIDGE Ⓥ

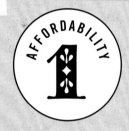

QUICK AND EASY TO MAKE, THIS BLEND OF
BUCKWHEAT, QUINOA AND MILLET FLAKES GIVES A
FINISHED PORRIDGE THAT HAS A SLIGHTLY SMOOTHER
TEXTURE THAN ONE MADE FROM ROLLED OATS.

1 Put the grain flakes, milk and water into a saucepan and
bring to the boil, then reduce the heat and cook for 4-5
minutes, stirring until thickened.

2 Mash 1 of the bananas and slice the other. Stir the mashed
banana into the porridge, then spoon into bowls and top
with spoonfuls of yogurt, the sliced banana, a drizzle of
honey or maple syrup and a sprinkling of cinnamon.
Serve immediately.

NUTRITIONAL TIP
Use unsweetened soya milk instead of dairy milk, if you prefer.
If you use soya yogurt rather than Greek yogurt, this dish will
be suitable for a dairy-free or vegan diet.

50 g (2 oz) buckwheat flakes
50 g (2 oz) quinoa flakes
50 g (2 oz) millet flakes
600 ml (1 pint) semi-skimmed milk
300 ml (½ pint) water
2 bananas, peeled

To serve
4 tablespoons 0%-fat Greek
yogurt
clear honey or maple syrup
sprinkling of ground cinnamon

Serves **4**
Prep time **5 minutes**
Cooking time **4-5 minutes**

PRUNE & BANANA CRUNCH Ⓥ

1 Mix together the banana, prunes and yogurt in a mixing bowl.

2 Spoon into 2 serving bowls and top with the cornflakes or crunchy cereal flakes. Serve immediately.

1 firm ripe banana, peeled and diced
100 g (3½ oz) ready-to-eat pitted dried prunes
250 ml (8 fl oz) 0%-fat Greek yogurt
40 g (1½ oz) cornflakes or crunchy cereal flakes

Serves **2**
Prep time **5 minutes**

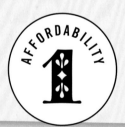

AFFORDABILITY
1

SPICED APPLE PORRIDGE

1 Put the apple juice and cinnamon in a microwave-proof serving bowl. Sprinkle in the millet flakes and stir gently.

2 Microwave on full power for 3-4 minutes, stirring frequently, until thick and creamy.

3 Alternatively, put the ingredients in a small saucepan and heat gently for 6-8 minutes, stirring frequently, until thick and creamy. Add a little extra juice if the mixture becomes dry.

4 Serve hot with the yogurt and, if you like your porridge sweet, a teaspoon or so of sugar.

VARIATION
For a berry compote, to serve with the granola instead of the fruit salad, place 150 g (5 oz) each of raspberries, blackberries and blueberries in a pan with the finely grated rind and juice of 1 lemon. Heat gently until the fruit has softened and the blueberries have burst, then sweeten with honey, to taste. Serve with the granola and yogurt, as above.

225 ml (7½ fl oz) apple juice
½ teaspoon ground cinnamon
25 g (1 oz) millet flakes

To serve
1 tablespoon 0%-fat Greek yogurt
demerara sugar (optional)

Serves **1**
Prep time **1 minute**
Cooking time **6-8 minutes**

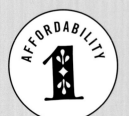

HEALTHY TIP

DON'T FLAG DOWN THE BUS If you live just a few stops from college there's no excuse not to walk. A brisk walk will get your heart pumping and your blood flowing — so you're less likely to doze off in the lecture theatre.

BANANA & SULTANA DROP SCONES (V)

1. Put the flour, sugar and baking powder in a mixing bowl. Add the mashed banana with the egg. Gradually whisk in the milk with a fork until the mixture resembles a smooth thick batter. Stir in the sultanas.

2. Pour a little oil on to a piece of folded kitchen paper and use to grease a griddle or heavy-based nonstick frying pan. Heat the pan, then drop heaped dessertspoonfuls of the mixture (in batches), well spaced apart, on to the pan. Cook for 2 minutes until bubbles appear on the top and the undersides are golden. Turn over and cook for a further 1-2 minutes until the second side is done.

3. Serve warm, topped with 1 teaspoon butter, honey, or golden or maple syrup per scone. These are best eaten on the day they are made.

VARIATION
For summer berry drop scones, prepare the recipe as above, but stir in 125 g (4 oz) mixed fresh blueberries and raspberries instead of the sultanas.

---

125 g (4 oz) self-raising flour
2 tablespoons caster sugar
½ teaspoon baking powder
1 small ripe banana, about 125 g (4 oz) with skin on, peeled and roughly mashed
1 egg, beaten
150 ml (¼ pint) milk
50 g (2 oz) sultanas
vegetable oil, for greasing
butter, clear honey, or golden or maple syrup, to serve

Makes **10**
Prep time **10 minutes**
Cooking time **8 minutes**

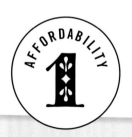
AFFORDABILITY
1

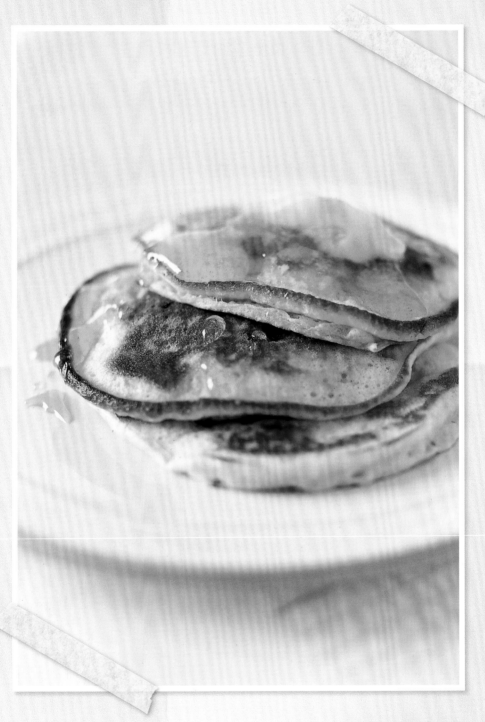

CORN & BACON MUFFINS

1 Lightly oil a 12-hole muffin tin.

2 Cut off any rind and excess fat, then finely chop the bacon and dry-fry it in a pan with the onion over a medium heat for 3–4 minutes until the bacon is turning crisp. Meanwhile, cook the sweetcorn in a small saucepan of boiling water for 2 minutes to soften, then drain.

3 Put the cornmeal, flour and baking powder in a bowl and mix together. Add the sweetcorn, bacon, onion and cheese and stir in.

4 Whisk the milk, eggs and oil together in a separate bowl or jug, then pour into the flour mixture and stir gently until just combined.

5 Divide the batter between the holes of the prepared muffin tin. Bake in a preheated oven, 220°C (425°F), Gas Mark 7, for 15–20 minutes until golden and just firm. Loosen the edges of the muffins with a knife and transfer to a wire rack to cool. Serve warm or cold. These are best eaten on the day they are made.

VARIATION
For spiced corn and spring onion muffins, omit the bacon. Prepare the recipe as above, replacing the red onion with 4 spring onions, thinly sliced into rounds, and add 1 teaspoon hot paprika and 1 deseeded and finely chopped red chilli to the mixture before baking.

3 tablespoons vegetable oil, plus extra for greasing
6 streaky bacon rashers
1 small red onion, finely chopped
200 g (7 oz) frozen sweetcorn
175 g (6 oz) fine cornmeal
125 g (4 oz) plain flour
2 teaspoons baking powder
50 g (2 oz) Cheddar cheese, grated
200 ml (7 fl oz) milk
2 eggs

Makes **12**
Prep time **15 minutes, plus cooling**
Cooking time **25 minutes**

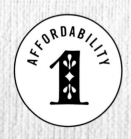

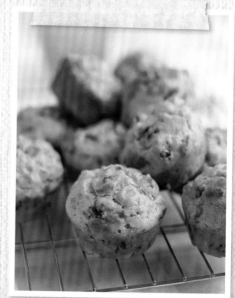

Very Berry MUFFINS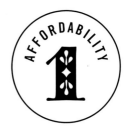

1 Line a 12-hole muffin tin with nonstick paper cases.

2 Put all the ingredients, except the berries, in a bowl and mix together to make a smooth batter. Fold in the berries.

3 Divide the mixture between the paper cases. Bake in a preheated oven, 180°C (350°F), Gas Mark 4, for 25 minutes or until a skewer comes out clean when inserted. Transfer to a wire rack to cool. Serve warm or cold. These are best eaten on the day they are made.

VARIATION

For banana and pecan muffins, prepare the recipe as above, but use 200 g (7 oz) chopped peeled bananas instead of the berries (select firm but ripe bananas), adding 125 g (4 oz) chopped pecan nuts with the bananas. Serve warm, drizzled with maple syrup, if liked.

250 g (8 oz) plain flour
4 tablespoons caster sugar
1 tablespoon baking powder
1 egg, beaten
200 ml (7 fl oz) milk
50 ml (2 fl oz) vegetable oil
200 g (7 oz) mixed fresh berries, roughly chopped

Makes **12**
Prep time **15 minutes, plus cooling**
Cooking time **25 minutes**

AFFORDABILITY 1

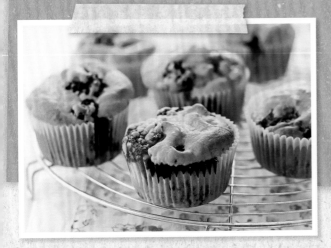

TRIPLE CHOCOLATE
PRETZELS

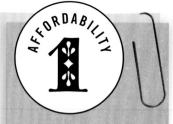

1 Oil 2 large baking sheets.

2 Mix the flour, yeast, sugar and salt in a mixing bowl. Add the melted butter or oil and gradually mix in the warm water until you have a smooth dough. Knead the dough for 5 minutes on a lightly floured surface until smooth and elastic.

3 Cut the dough into quarters, then cut each quarter into 10 smaller pieces. Shape each piece into a thin rope about 20 cm (8 inches) long. Bend each rope so that it forms a wide arc, then bring one of the ends round in a loop and secure about halfway along the rope. Do the same with the other end, looping it across the first secured end. Repeat with all the pieces of dough.

4 Transfer the pretzels to the prepared baking sheets. Cover loosely with lightly oiled clingfilm and leave in a warm place for 30 minutes until well risen.

5 Make the glaze. Mix the water and salt in a bowl until the salt has dissolved, then brush this over the pretzels. Bake in a preheated oven, 200°C (400°F), Gas Mark 6, for 6-8 minutes until golden brown. Transfer to a wire rack to cool.

6 Melt the different chocolates in 3 separate heatproof bowls set over saucepans of barely simmering water. Drizzle random lines of dark chocolate over the pretzels, using a spoon. Leave to harden, then repeat with the white and then the milk chocolate. Store in an airtight tin for up to 2 days.

VARIATION
For classic pretzels, brush plain pretzels as soon as they come out of the oven with a glaze made by heating 2 teaspoons salt, ½ teaspoon caster sugar and 2 tablespoons water in a saucepan until dissolved.

vegetable oil, for greasing
225 g (7½ oz) strong white flour, plus extra for dusting
1 teaspoon fast-action dried yeast
2 teaspoons caster sugar
large pinch of salt
15 g (½ oz) butter, melted, or 1 tablespoon sunflower oil
125 ml (4 fl oz) hand-hot water
75 g (3 oz) each plain dark, white and milk chocolate, broken into pieces

Glaze
2 tablespoons water
½ teaspoon salt

Makes **40**
Prep time **30 minutes, plus rising, cooling and setting**
Cooking time **15 minutes**

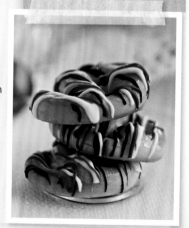

Fruited
GRIDDLE CAKES Ⓥ

1 Put the flour in a mixing bowl or a food processor. Add the butter and rub in with your fingertips, or process until the mixture resembles fine breadcrumbs. Stir in the sugar, dried fruit, spice and lemon rind. Add the egg, then gradually mix in the milk, if needed, to make a smooth dough.

2 Knead the dough lightly, then roll out on a lightly floured surface until 5 mm (¼ inch) thick. Stamp out 5 cm (2 inch) rounds using a fluted round biscuit cutter or a glass. Re-knead the trimmings and continue rolling and stamping out until all the dough has been used.

3 Pour a little oil on to a piece of folded kitchen paper and use to grease a griddle or heavy-based nonstick frying pan. Heat the pan, then add the cakes in batches, re-greasing the griddle or pan as needed, and fry over a medium-low heat for about 3 minutes on each side until golden brown and cooked through.

4 Serve warm, sprinkled with a little extra sugar or spread with butter, if liked. Store in an airtight tin for up to 2 days.

VARIATION
For orange and cinnamon griddle cakes, prepare the recipe as above, but use the finely grated rind of ½ orange instead of the lemon, and 1 teaspoon ground cinnamon in place of the mixed spice.

250 g (8 oz) self-raising flour, plus extra for dusting
125 g (4 oz) butter, diced, plus extra for spreading
100 g (3½ oz) caster sugar, plus extra for sprinkling
50 g (2 oz) currants
50 g (2 oz) sultanas
1 teaspoon ground mixed spice
finely grated rind of ½ lemon
1 egg, beaten
1 tablespoon milk, if needed
vegetable oil, for greasing

Serves **30**
Prep time **25 minutes**
Cooking time **18 minutes**

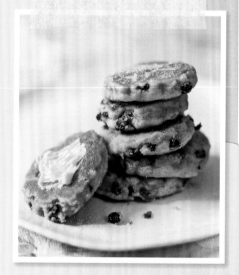

Porridge with Prune Compote (V)

1 Place all the compote ingredients in a small saucepan over a medium heat. Simmer gently for 10-12 minutes or until softened and slightly sticky. Leave to cool. (The compote can be prepared in advance and chilled. Remember to remove the cinnamon stick and clove before serving.)

2 Put the milk, water, vanilla extract, cinnamon and salt in a large saucepan over a medium heat and bring slowly to the boil. Stir in the oats, then reduce the heat and simmer gently, stirring occasionally, for 8-10 minutes until creamy and tender.

3 Spoon the porridge into bowls, scatter with the almonds and serve with the prune compote.

VARIATION
For sweet quinoa porridge with banana and dates, put 250 g (8 oz) quinoa in a saucepan with the milk, 1 tablespoon agave nectar or clear honey and 2-3 cardamom pods, crushed. Simmer gently for 12-15 minutes or until the quinoa is cooked and the desired consistency is reached. Discard the cardamom pods. Serve the porridge in bowls topped with a dollop of natural yogurt, 100 g (3½ oz) chopped pitted dates and sliced banana.

1 litre (1¾ pints) skimmed or semi-skimmed milk
500 ml (17 fl oz) water
1 teaspoon vanilla extract
pinch of ground cinnamon
pinch of salt
200 g (7 oz) porridge oats
3 tablespoons flaked almonds, toasted

Compote
250 g (8 oz) ready-to-eat pitted dried Agen prunes
125 ml (4 fl oz) apple juice
1 small cinnamon stick
1 whole clove
1 tablespoon clear honey
1 unpeeled orange quarter

Serves **8**
Prep time **5 minutes**
Cooking time **20-25 minutes**

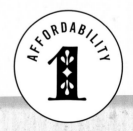
AFFORDABILITY 1

Wholemeal
BLUEBERRY PANCAKES
WITH LEMON CURD YOGURT

1 Sift the flours and baking powder into a large bowl, then make a well in the centre. Mix together the milk, egg and honey in a jug, then pour into the dry ingredients and whisk until mixed. Stir in 150 g (5 oz) of the blueberries.

2 Heat the coconut oil in a large frying pan, then drop 2 tablespoons of the batter into the pan for each pancake to form 4 and cook for 4-5 minutes until golden, then turn over and cook for a further 2-3 minutes. Remove from the pan and keep warm. Repeat with the remaining batter to make about 12.

3 Mix together the lemon curd and yogurt in a small bowl. Serve the warm pancakes with dollops of the lemon yogurt, sprinkled with the remaining blueberries and drizzled with honey.

150 g (5 oz) wholemeal plain flour
50 g (2 oz) plain flour
1 teaspoon baking powder
300 ml (½ pint) milk
1 egg, beaten
2 tablespoons clear honey, plus extra for drizzling
175 g (6 oz) blueberries
25 g (1 oz) coconut oil
1 tablespoon lemon curd
125 ml (4 fl oz) natural yogurt

Serves **4**
Prep time **15 minutes**
Cooking time **25 minutes**

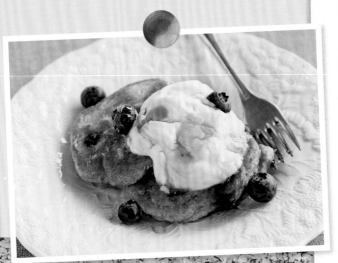

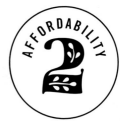

AFFORDABILITY

HEALTHY LUNCHES
and snacks

Buying lunches and snacks in the college canteen every day can put a serious dent in your finances. Equally, you're more likely to plump for the unhealthy option when you're in a hurry and need a quick fix for a rumbling stomach. But if you can get organized and give yourself an extra 5 minutes in the morning, it's easy to throw together a healthy lunch that will keep you going through the afternoon and leave you money to spare at the end of the week.

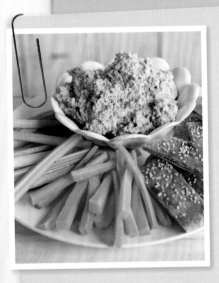

LOVE YOUR LEFTOVERS

Surely the quickest lunch of all – just make a little extra when you're cooking dinner and pop a serving in a container for the next day. This is ideal for pasta, noodles and rice dishes. Alternatively, if you're cooking pasta for dinner, you could double the amount of pasta; use what you need for your main meal, then allow the rest to cool and stir through green or red pesto and lunch is sorted.

VEGETABLE PLATTER

Slice up a bundle of crudités (cucumber, celery, carrot, pepper, cauliflower) and cut a pitta bread into thin strips. Pack in a plastic container with a mini hummus pot.

GOING GREEN

You can make a salad out of pretty much anything – start with the obvious salad leaves, tomato, cucumber and celery, and liven it up with leftover cooked meat, canned fish, pulses, peppers and a simple homemade dressing of olive oil and balsamic vinegar.

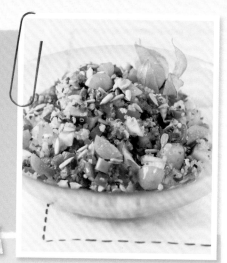

WINTER WARMER

A flask or thermos is a good investment for your kitchen. If you make a big batch of soup (see recipes on pages 48–55), you'll have enough lunches for a week. Heat up the amount you need and pour into a flask, then grab a roll or a couple of slices of buttered bread to make a meal of it.

IT'S A WRAP

Wraps are cheap, healthy and versatile. Try these fillings:
- COOKED CHICKEN & PESTO
- CREAM CHEESE, GRATED CARROT & LETTUCE
- FALAFEL & HUMMUS
- TUNA, MAYONNAISE & KIDNEY BEANS
- CHICKPEAS WITH CHOPPED RED PEPPER & CUCUMBER

AN EGGCELLENT IDEA

Tortilla is healthy, filling and quick to make. Fry a chopped onion in a medium frying pan. Add some chopped deseeded red or yellow pepper and courgette, cooked diced potato, crushed garlic and chopped tomato. Pour in 4 beaten eggs and cook, stirring. As the eggs start to set, cook for another minute or so, then finish off under a preheated hot grill for 1–2 minutes. Place a plate over the pan and tip it over so the tortilla lands on the plate. Leave to cool, then divide into large slices for lunch over the next couple of days or so. See page 72 for an alternative tasty Spinach & Potato Tortilla recipe.

ON-THE-GO
Granola Breakfast Bars

1 Grease a shallow 20 cm (8 inch) square tin.

2 Place the butter and honey in a saucepan and bring gently to the boil, stirring continuously, until the mixture bubbles. Add the cinnamon, dried fruit, seeds and nuts, then stir and heat for 1 minute.

3 Remove from the heat and add the oats. Stir well, then transfer to the prepared tin and press down well. Bake in a preheated oven, 190°C (375°F), Gas Mark 5, for 15 minutes until the top is just beginning to brown.

4 Leave to cool in the tin, then cut into 9 squares or bars to serve. Store in an airtight tin for up to 2 days.

75 g (3 oz) butter, plus extra
  for greasing
75 ml (3 fl oz) clear honey
½ teaspoon ground cinnamon
100 g (3½ oz) ready-to-eat dried
  apricots, roughly chopped
50 g (2 oz) ready-to-eat dried
  papaya or mango, roughly
  chopped
50 g (2 oz) raisins
4 tablespoons mixed seeds,
  such as pumpkin, sesame
  and sunflower
50 g (2 oz) pecan nuts, roughly
  broken
150 g (5 oz) porridge oats

Makes **9**
Prep time **15 minutes, plus cooling**
Cooking time **15 minutes**

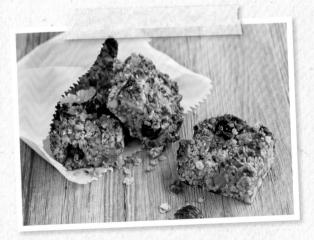

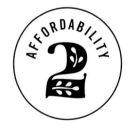

AFFORDABILITY
2

FRUITY MANGO FLAPJACKS Ⓥ

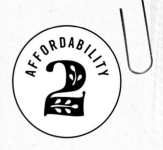

1 Place the sugar, butter and syrup in a heavy-based saucepan and heat gently until melted, then stir in the remaining ingredients until combined.

2 Spoon the mixture into a 28 x 18 cm (11 x 7 inch) nonstick baking tin lined with baking paper and press down lightly. Bake in a preheated oven, 150°C (300°F), Gas Mark 2, for 30 minutes or until pale golden brown.

3 Mark into 12 pieces, then cool before removing from the tin. Cut or break into pieces to serve. Store in an airtight tin for up to 2 days.

VARIATION

For honey and ginger flapjacks, place 50 g (2 oz) soft light brown sugar in a saucepan with 50 g (2 oz) clear honey and the butter. Omit the golden syrup. Heat until melted, then add the millet flakes or 200 g (7 oz) porridge oats and the seeds. Instead of the dried mango, stir in 1 ball of preserved stem ginger, drained and finely chopped. Spoon the mixture into the tin and complete the recipe as above.

100 g (3½ oz) soft light brown sugar
150 g (5 oz) butter
2 tablespoons golden syrup
200 g (7 oz) millet flakes
2 tablespoons mixed seeds, such as pumpkin and sunflower
75 g (3 oz) ready-to-eat dried mango, roughly chopped

Makes **12**
Prep time **10 minutes, plus cooling**
Cooking time **30 minutes**

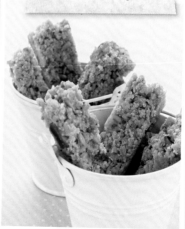

SEEDED SPELT SODA BREAD (V)

1 Grease a loaf tin with a capacity of at least 750 ml (1¼ pints). If you don't have a loaf tin, grease a baking sheet.

2 Sift the flours and baking powder into a bowl. Tip in the grain left in the sieve and stir in the salt and seeds. Add the buttermilk and milk and mix with a round-bladed knife to form a soft dough.

3 Turn out on to a lightly floured surface and shape into an oblong. Turn into the prepared tin or neaten the shape and place on the baking sheet. Bake in a preheated oven, 200°C (400°F), Gas Mark 6, for 20 minutes.

4 Reduce the oven temperature to 160°C (325°F), Gas Mark 3, and bake for a further 15 minutes. Turn out of the tin (if using) and return to the oven shelf for a further 10 minutes baking. Leave to cool completely on a wire rack. Serve in slices. This is best eaten on the day it is made.

vegetable oil, for greasing
250 g (8 oz) spelt flour, plus extra for dusting
100 g (3½ oz) rye flour
2 teaspoons baking powder
1 teaspoon salt
40 g (1½ oz) pumpkin seeds
40 g (1½ oz) sunflower seeds
284 ml (9½ fl oz) carton buttermilk
100 ml (3½ fl oz) semi-skimmed milk

Makes **1 loaf; serves 8**
Prep time **10 minutes, plus cooling**
Cooking time **45 minutes**

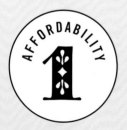
AFFORDABILITY
1

STUDENT TIP

BREADCRUMBS When you get to the last slice of bread, don't throw it away if it's a bit dry — blitz it in a blender and keep the breadcrumbs in an airtight container in the freezer. They're great for pie and bake toppings.

FALAFEL PITTA POCKETS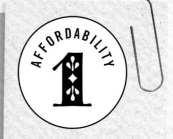

1 Put the chickpeas in a bowl, add cold water to cover by a generous 10 cm (4 inches) and leave to soak overnight.

2 Drain the chickpeas, transfer to a blender or food processor and process until coarsely ground. Add the onion, garlic, fresh herbs, ground coriander and baking powder. Season with salt and pepper and process until really smooth. Using wet hands, shape the mixture into 16 small patties.

3 Heat the oil in a large frying pan over a medium-high heat, add the patties, in batches, and fry for 3 minutes on each side or until golden and cooked through. Remove with a slotted spoon and drain on kitchen paper.

4 Split the pitta breads and fill with the falafel, salad leaves and diced tomatoes. Add a spoonful of the yogurt to each and serve immediately.

VARIATION
For a falafel salad, toss 4 handfuls of mixed salad leaves with a little olive oil, lemon juice and salt and pepper and arrange on serving plates. Core, deseed and dice 1 red pepper and sprinkle it over the salads. Top with the falafel and spoon over a little natural or 0%-fat Greek yogurt.

250 g (8 oz) dried chickpeas
1 small onion, finely chopped
2 garlic cloves, crushed
½ bunch of parsley
½ bunch of fresh coriander
2 teaspoons ground coriander
½ teaspoon baking powder
2 tablespoons vegetable oil
4 wholemeal pitta breads
handful of salad leaves
2 tomatoes, diced
4 tablespoons 0%-fat Greek yogurt
salt and pepper

Serves **4**
Prep time **15 minutes, plus overnight soaking**
Cooking time **12 minutes**

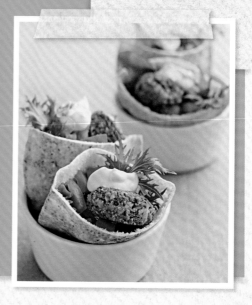

FALAFELS WITH BEETROOT SALAD & MINT YOGURT

1 To make the falafels, place the chickpeas, onion, garlic, chilli, cumin, coriander and parsley in a blender or food processor. Season with salt and pepper, then process to make a coarse paste. Shape the mixture into 8 patties and set aside.

2 To make the salad, place the carrot, beetroot and spinach in a bowl. Season with salt and pepper, add the lemon juice and oil and stir well.

3 To make the mint yogurt, mix all the ingredients together in a small bowl and season with a little salt.

4 Heat the oil in a frying pan, add the falafels and fry for 4-5 minutes on each side until golden. Serve with the beetroot salad and mint yogurt.

Falafels
400 g (13 oz) can chickpeas, rinsed and drained
½ small red onion, roughly chopped
1 garlic clove, chopped
½ red chilli, deseeded
1 teaspoon ground cumin
1 teaspoon ground coriander
handful of flat leaf parsley
2 tablespoons olive oil
salt and pepper

Beetroot salad
1 carrot, coarsely grated
1 raw beetroot, coarsely grated
50 g (2 oz) baby spinach leaves
1 tablespoon lemon juice
2 tablespoons olive oil

Mint yogurt
150 ml (¼ pint) 0%-fat Greek yogurt
1 tablespoon chopped mint leaves
½ garlic clove, crushed

Serves **2**
Prep time **20 minutes**
Cooking time **10 minutes**

AFFORDABILITY
1

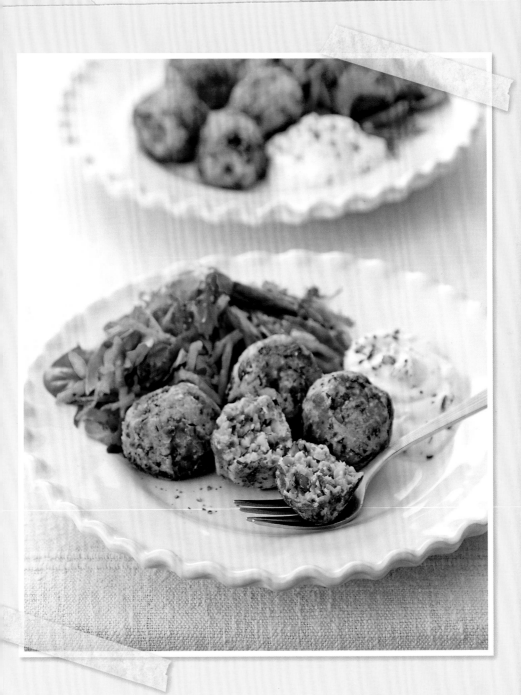

brown rice salad
WITH PEANUTS & RAISINS

1 Cook the rice in a saucepan of lightly salted boiling water for 15-18 minutes until tender.

2 Meanwhile, place the spring onions, raisins, red pepper and peanuts in a large bowl and toss with the soy sauce and oil until well coated.

3 Once the rice is cooked, drain it in a sieve and rinse with cold water until cold. Once cold and drained, add to the other ingredients and toss well to coat and mix.

4 Turn into a serving bowl and serve, or place in a lunch box with slices of cheese or meat to serve alongside, if liked.

200 g (7 oz) easy-cook brown rice
bunch of spring onions, roughly chopped
125 g (4 oz) raisins
1 red pepper, cored, deseeded and sliced
75 g (3 oz) roasted peanuts
2 tablespoons dark soy sauce
1 tablespoon sesame oil
salt

Serves **4**
Prep time **10 minutes**
Cooking time **18 minutes**

AFFORDABILITY
1

HEALTHY TIP

GO NUTS FOR NUTS The ultimate healthy snack but nuts can be quite pricey so buy a huge pack and divide it into smaller portions and you'll save money. Go for unsalted/unflavoured (natural) nuts and don't forget seeds (such as sunflower, pumpkin and linseeds) – a healthy snack and great for sprinkling.

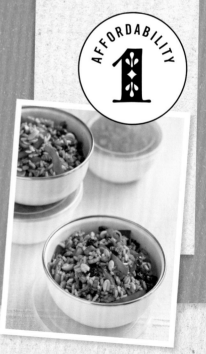

PORK & APPLE BALLS

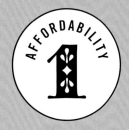
1 Place the apple and onion in a bowl with the minced pork and, using a fork, mash all the ingredients together well. Shape into 16 rough balls. Place the breadcrumbs on a plate and roll the balls in the breadcrumbs to lightly coat all over.

2 Heat the oil in a large, heavy-based frying pan and cook the pork balls over a medium-high heat for 8–10 minutes, turning frequently, until cooked through. Drain on kitchen paper.

3 Serve warm with tomato chutney and cherry tomatoes, and provide bamboo paddle skewers or forks for dipping the balls in the chutney.

1 small dessert apple, such as Cox's, cored and grated (with skin on)
1 small onion, grated
250 g (8 oz) minced pork
50 g (2 oz) wholemeal breadcrumbs
3 tablespoons vegetable oil

To serve
tomato chutney
cherry tomatoes

Serves **4**
Prep time **15 minutes**
Cooking time **10 minutes**

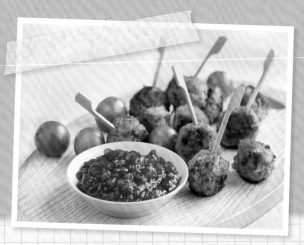

Sweet Potato & Bean 'STEAMED BUNS'

1. Mix the grated courgette with the sugar and 2 teaspoons of the vinegar in a small bowl and leave to stand while preparing the filling.

2. Thinly slice the sweet potatoes and cook in a saucepan of boiling water for 8-10 minutes until just tender. Add the beans and cook for a further 2 minutes to soften. Drain.

3. Add the hoisin sauce and the remaining vinegar to the saucepan. Tip in the drained vegetables, spring onions and coriander and mix well.

4. Wrap the pitta breads in clingfilm and microwave on full power for 1-2 minutes until soft.

5. Split the pittas and fill with the sweet potato mixture. Spoon the courgette mixture on top, then serve.

100 g (3½ oz) courgette, coarsely grated
1 teaspoon caster sugar
3 teaspoons rice vinegar
300 g (10 oz) sweet potatoes, scrubbed
100 g (3½ oz) French beans, trimmed and cut into 2.5 cm (1 inch) lengths
50 ml (2 fl oz) hoisin sauce
4 spring onions, thinly sliced
4 tablespoons chopped fresh coriander
2 wholemeal or white pitta breads

Serves **2**
Prep time **15 minutes**
Cooking time **14 minutes**

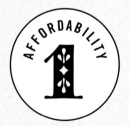

TUNA & SWEETCORN WRAPS

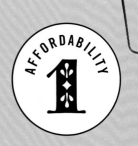

1 Place the eggs in a saucepan of water and bring to the boil. Reduce the heat and simmer for 10 minutes until hard-boiled. Remove from the pan and plunge into cold water to cool.

2 Meanwhile, place the tuna and sweetcorn in a mixing bowl and season with pepper. Add the mayonnaise and mix together.

3 Lay the tortillas or chapattis on a chopping board and divide the tuna mixture between them, piling it across the middle of each. Shell the eggs and roughly chop, then scatter over the tuna mixture. Scatter with the cress. Sprinkle each with a pinch of paprika, then roll up tightly and cut in half to serve. Wrap in greaseproof paper to travel, if liked.

2 eggs
400 g (13 oz) can tuna, drained
75 g (3 oz) canned sweetcorn, drained, or frozen sweetcorn
4 tablespoons mayonnaise
4 wholemeal soft flour tortillas or thin chapattis
1 punnet of cress, cut
4 pinches of paprika
pepper

Serves **4**
Prep time **15 minutes**
Cooking time **15 minutes**

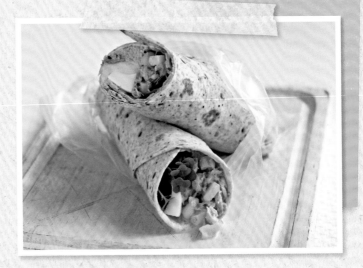

Mushroom & Rocket
SEEDED WRAP
WITH FETA & GARLIC DRESSING

1   Crumble the feta into a small bowl and stir in the yogurt.
    Season with plenty of pepper and beat well with a fork.

2   Heat the oil in a small frying pan and fry the mushrooms
    for about 5 minutes until beginning to colour and the juices
    have evaporated. Stir in the garam masala and a pinch of
    salt and cook for a further 2 minutes.

3   Lightly grill the wrap under a preheated hot grill until
    warmed through. Spread with the feta mixture and tip the
    mushrooms on top. Scatter with the beans and rocket and
    drizzle with the honey. Roll up loosely to serve.

40 g (1½ oz) feta cheese
50 ml (2 fl oz) 0%-fat Greek
   yogurt
1 tablespoon oil
200 g (7 oz) mushrooms, trimmed
   and thinly sliced
½ teaspoon garam masala
1 seeded wrap
25 g (1 oz) sprouting beans
small handful of rocket, about 15 g
   (½ oz)
1 teaspoon clear honey
salt and pepper

Serves **1**
Prep time **5 minutes**
Cooking time **8 minutes**

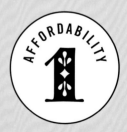

BLACKENED TOFU WRAPS (V)

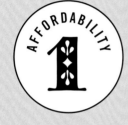

AFFORDABILITY 1

200 g (7 oz) tofu
1 tablespoon dark muscovado sugar
1 teaspoon pepper
1 teaspoon five-spice powder
½ teaspoon ground ginger
1 garlic clove, crushed
2 seeded wraps
2 tablespoons sesame oil
50 g (2 oz) mixed salad leaves
1 carrot, grated
½ bunch of spring onions, thinly sliced
1 tablespoon clear honey
squeeze of lime or lemon juice
salt

Serves **2**
Prep time **10 minutes**
Cooking time **5 minutes**

1 Thoroughly drain the tofu between several sheets of kitchen paper. Cut into thin slices. Mix together the sugar, pepper, five-spice powder, ginger and a little salt. Spread the garlic over the tofu, then dust on both sides with the spice mixture.

2 Warm the wraps in a frying pan or under a preheated hot grill.

3 Heat 1 tablespoon of the oil in a frying pan and fry the tofu slices for 1–2 minutes on each side until deep golden.

4 Scatter the salad leaves, carrot and spring onions over the warm wraps, then place the tofu slices on top, placing them over the length of the wraps.

5 Add the remaining oil, the honey and lime or lemon juice to the pan and stir to mix. Drizzle over the wraps, roll and then serve warm or cold.

Healthy & Hearty

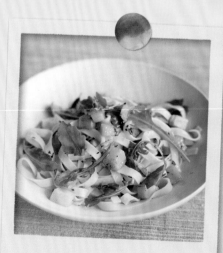

TAGLIATELLE WITH PUMPKIN & SAGE

HEARTY
MINESTRONE

1 Whizz the carrots, onion and celery in a blender or food processor until finely chopped.

2 Heat the oil in a large saucepan, add the chopped vegetables, garlic, potatoes, tomato purée, stock, tomatoes and pasta. Bring to the boil, then reduce the heat and simmer, covered, for 12-15 minutes, stirring occasionally.

3 Tip in the cannellini beans and the spinach for the final 2 minutes of the cooking time.

4 Season to taste with salt and pepper and serve with crusty bread.

3 carrots, roughly chopped
1 red onion, roughly chopped
6 celery sticks, roughly chopped
2 tablespoons olive oil
2 garlic cloves, crushed
200 g (7 oz) potatoes, peeled and cut into 1 cm (½ inch) dice
4 tablespoons tomato purée
1.5 litres (2½ pints) Vegetable Stock (see page 244)
400 g (13 oz) can chopped tomatoes
150 g (5 oz) short-shaped soup pasta
400 g (13 oz) can cannellini beans, rinsed and drained
100 g (3½ oz) baby spinach
salt and pepper
crusty bread, to serve

Serves **4**
Prep time **10 minutes**
Cooking time **20 minutes**

HEALTHY TIP

WISE UP TO WATER It really is the elixir of life so try to make sure you drink more aqua than alcohol. Keep a bottle in your bag and drink regularly throughout the day to keep your brain alert and lethargy at bay.

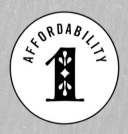

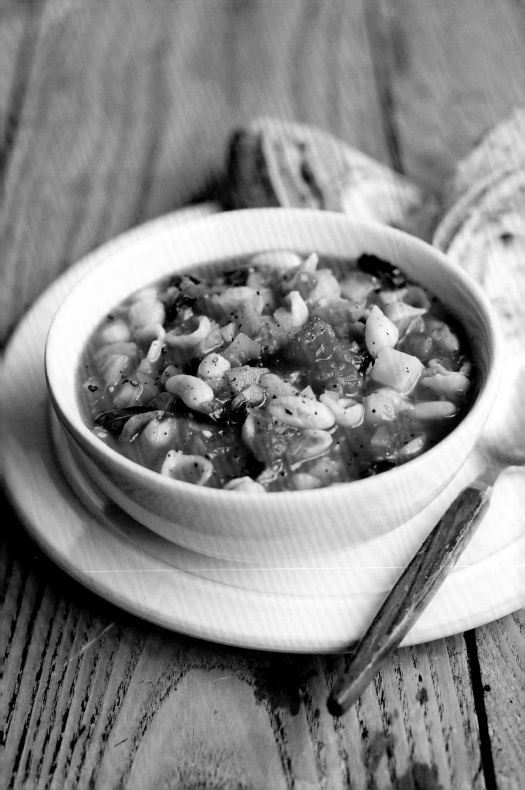

Summer
VEGETABLE SOUP

1 Heat the oil in a medium saucepan and fry the leek for 3-4 minutes until softened. Add the potato and stock to the pan and cook for 10 minutes. Add the mixed summer vegetables and the mint, then bring to the boil. Reduce the heat and simmer, stirring occasionally, for 10 minutes.

2 Cool slightly, then transfer the soup to a blender or food processor and purée until smooth. Return the soup to the pan, add the crème fraîche and season to taste with salt and pepper. Heat through gently and serve.

VARIATION

For chunky summer vegetable soup with mixed herb gremolata, make up the soup as above but do not purée. Ladle the soup into bowls and serve topped with 2 tablespoons of crème fraîche and gremolata, made by mixing together 2 tablespoons chopped basil, 2 tablespoons chopped parsley, the finely grated rind of 1 lemon and 1 finely chopped small garlic clove.

1 teaspoon olive oil
1 leek, trimmed, cleaned and thinly sliced
1 large potato, peeled and chopped
900 ml (1½ pints) Vegetable Stock (see page 244)
450 g (14½ oz) prepared mixed summer vegetables (such as peas, asparagus, broad beans and courgettes)
2 tablespoons chopped mint
2 tablespoons half-fat crème fraîche
salt and pepper

Serves **4**
Prep time **15 minutes**
Cooking time **30 minutes**

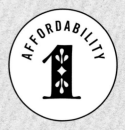

RED PEPPER & COURGETTE SOUP

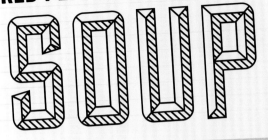

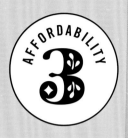

1 Heat the oil in a large saucepan and gently fry the onions for 5 minutes or until softened and golden brown. Add the garlic and cook gently for 1 minute. Add the red peppers and half of the courgettes to the pan. Fry for 5-8 minutes or until softened and brown.

2 Add the stock to the pan, season to taste with salt and pepper and bring to the boil. Reduce the heat, cover the pan and simmer gently, stirring occasionally, for 20 minutes.

3 Allow the soup to cool slightly once the vegetables are tender, then purée in batches in a blender or food processor. Gently fry the remaining chopped courgettes for 5 minutes (you may need to add a little more oil to the pan).

4 Meanwhile, return the soup to the pan, reheat gently, then taste and adjust the seasoning if needed. Serve topped with the fried courgettes, yogurt or crème fraîche and chives.

VARIATION

For red pepper and carrot soup, make up the soup as above, adding 2 diced carrots instead of the courgettes, plus the red peppers, to the fried onion and garlic. Continue as above. Purée, reheat and serve topped with teaspoonfuls of garlic and herb soft cheese and some snipped chives.

2 tablespoons olive oil
2 onions, finely chopped
1 garlic clove, crushed
3 red peppers, cored, deseeded and roughly chopped
2 courgettes, roughly chopped
900 ml (1½ pints) Vegetable Stock (see page 244)
salt and pepper

To serve
low-fat natural yogurt or half-fat crème fraîche
whole chives

Serves **4**
Prep time **15 minutes**
Cooking time **40 minutes**

BEEF
& BARLEY BRÖ

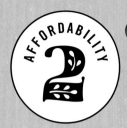

AFFORDABILITY **2**

1 Melt the butter in a large saucepan, then add the beef and onion and fry for 5 minutes, stirring, until the beef is browned and the onion is just beginning to colour.

2 Stir in the diced vegetables, pearl barley, stock and mustard, if using. Season with salt and pepper and bring to the boil. Cover and simmer for 1¾ hours, stirring occasionally, until the meat and vegetables are very tender. Taste and adjust the seasoning if needed.

3 Ladle the soup into bowls and sprinkle with a little chopped parsley just before serving.

VARIATION
For a lamb and barley hotchpot, substitute the beef for 250 g (8 oz) diced lamb fillet and fry with the onion as above. Add the sliced white part of 1 trimmed and cleaned leek, 175 g (6 oz) each of diced swede, carrot and potato, hen mix in 50 g (2 oz) pearl barley, 2 litres (3½ pints) lamb stock, 2-3 sprigs of rosemary and salt and pepper. Bring to the boil, then cover and simmer for 1¾ hours. Discard the rosemary, add the remaining thinly sliced green leek and cook for a further 10 minutes. Ladle into bowls and sprinkle with a little extra chopped rosemary to serve.

25 g (1 oz) butter
250 g (8 oz) braising beef, fat trimmed away and meat cut into small cubes
1 large onion, finely chopped
200 g (7 oz) swede, diced
150 g (5 oz) carrot, diced
100 g (3½ oz) pearl barley
2 litres (3½ pints) beef stock
2 teaspoons dry English mustard (optional)
salt and pepper
chopped parsley, to garnish

Serves **6**
Prep time **20 minutes**
Cooking time **1¾ hours**

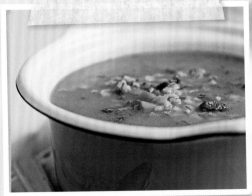

BUTTERNUT & ROSEMARY SOUP

1. Place the squash pieces in a nonstick roasting tin. Sprinkle over the rosemary sprigs and season with salt and pepper. Roast in a preheated oven, 200°C (400°F), Gas Mark 6, for 45 minutes.

2. Meanwhile, put the lentils in a saucepan and cover with water, then bring to the boil and boil rapidly for 10 minutes. Drain, then return to a clean saucepan with the onion and stock and simmer for 5 minutes. Season with salt and pepper.

3. Remove the squash from the oven and scoop the flesh from the skin. Mash the flesh with a fork and add it to the soup, then simmer for 25 minutes, stirring occasionally, until the lentils are tender. Serve the soup scattered with extra rosemary.

1 butternut squash, halved, deseeded and cut into small chunks
few rosemary sprigs, plus extra leaves to garnish
150 g (5 oz) red lentils, rinsed and drained
1 onion, finely chopped
900 ml (1½ pints) Vegetable Stock (see page 244)
salt and pepper

Serves **4**
Prep time **15 minutes**
Cooking time **1 hour 10 minutes**

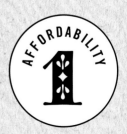

SQUASH, KALE & MIXED BEAN SOUP (V)

1 Heat the oil in a saucepan over a medium-low heat, add the onion and fry gently for 5 minutes. Stir in the garlic and smoked paprika and cook briefly, then add the squash, carrots, tomatoes and mixed beans. Pour in the stock, season with salt and pepper and bring to the boil, stirring frequently. Reduce the heat, cover and simmer for 25 minutes, stirring occasionally, until the vegetables are cooked and tender.

2 Stir in the crème fraîche, then add the kale, pressing it just beneath the surface of the stock. Cover and cook for 5 minutes or until the kale has just wilted. Ladle into bowls and serve with warm garlic bread, if liked.

VARIATION
For cheesy squash, pepper and mixed bean soup, make as above, replacing the carrots with 1 cored, deseeded and diced red pepper. Pour in the stock, then add 65 g (2½ oz) Parmesan-style cheese rinds and season. Cover and simmer for 25 minutes. Stir in the crème fraîche but omit the kale. Discard the cheese rinds, ladle the soup into bowls and top with grated Parmesan-style cheese.

1 tablespoon olive oil
1 onion, finely chopped
2 garlic cloves, finely chopped
1 teaspoon smoked paprika
500 g (1 lb) butternut squash, halved, deseeded, peeled and diced
2 small carrots, peeled and diced
500 g (1 lb) tomatoes, skinned (optional) and roughly chopped
400 g (13 oz) can mixed beans, rinsed and drained
900 ml (1½ pints) Vegetable Stock (see page 244)
150 ml (¼ pint) half-fat crème fraîche
100 g (3½ oz) kale, torn into bite-sized pieces
salt and pepper
crusty bread or warm garlic bread, to serve (optional)

Serves **6**
Prep time **15 minutes**
Cooking time **45 minutes**

AFFORDABILITY 1

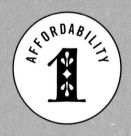

Sweet Potato & CABBAGE SOUP

1 Place the onions, garlic and bacon in a large saucepan and fry for 2–3 minutes. Add the sweet potatoes, parsnips, thyme and stock, then bring to the boil and simmer for 15 minutes, stirring occasionally.

2 Cool slightly, then transfer two-thirds of the soup to a blender or food processor and blend until smooth. Return to the pan, add the cabbage and simmer for 5–7 minutes until the cabbage is just cooked. Serve with Irish soda bread.

VARIATION
For squash and broccoli soup, follow the recipe above, replacing the sweet potatoes with 500 g (1 lb) peeled, deseeded and chopped butternut squash. After returning the blended soup to the pan, add 100 g (3½ oz) small broccoli florets. Cook as above, omitting the cabbage.

2 onions, chopped
2 garlic cloves, sliced
4 lean back bacon rashers, chopped
500 g (1 lb) sweet potatoes, scrubbed or peeled and chopped
2 parsnips, chopped
1 teaspoon chopped thyme
900 ml (1½ pints) Vegetable Stock (see page 244)
1 baby Savoy cabbage, shredded
Irish soda bread, to serve

Serves **4**
Prep time **15 minutes**
Cooking time **25 minutes**

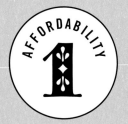

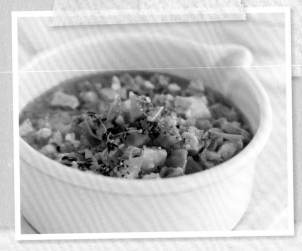

TAGLIATELLE
WITH PUMPKIN & SAGE

1 Place the pumpkin into a small roasting tin, add 2 tablespoons of the oil, season with salt and pepper and toss to mix well. Roast in a preheated oven, 220°C (425°F), Gas Mark 7, for 15-20 minutes or until just tender.

2 Meanwhile, bring a large saucepan of lightly salted water to the boil. Cook the pasta according to the packet instructions.

3 Drain the pasta, return to the pan, then add the rocket, sage and roasted pumpkin. Mix together over a gentle heat with the remaining oil until the rocket has wilted, then serve with a good grating of cheese, if liked.

875 g (1¾ lb) pumpkin, butternut
  or winter squash, peeled,
  deseeded and cut into 1.5 cm
  (¾ inch) cubes
4 tablespoons olive oil
500 g (1 lb) fresh tagliatelle
50 g (2 oz) rocket
8 sage leaves, chopped
salt and pepper
grated Parmesan-style cheese,
  to serve (optional)

Makes **4**
Prep time **15 minutes**
Cooking time **15-20 minutes**

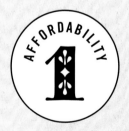

STUDENT TIP

COMPARE PRICES Every penny counts when you're shopping on a budget so try out a price comparison site to make sure you're getting the best supermarket deals in your basket.

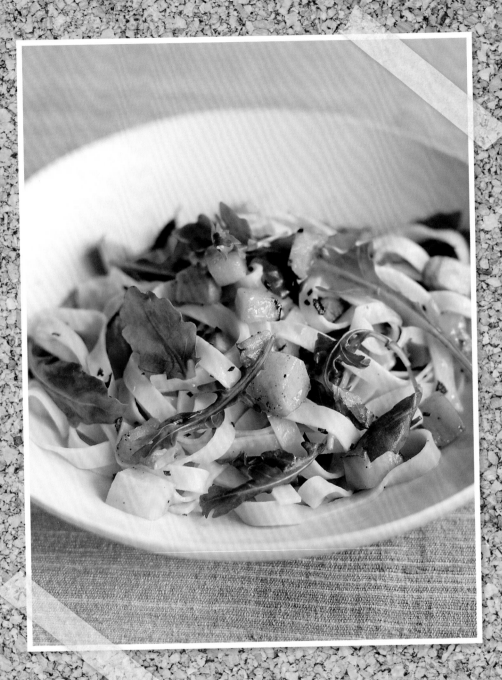

Aubergine
CANNELLONI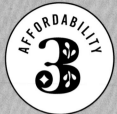

ALTHOUGH A LITTLE FIDDLY TO PREPARE, THIS DISH IS WELL WORTH THE EFFORT, MAKING A DELICIOUS COMBINATION OF CREAMY RICOTTA FILLING AND SWEET, GRILLED AUBERGINES.

1 Bring a saucepan of lightly salted water to the boil. Add the lasagne sheets, return to the boil and cook, allowing 2 minutes for fresh and 8-10 minutes for dried. Drain the sheets and immerse in cold water.

2 Place the aubergine slices in a single layer on a foil-lined grill rack. (You may need to do this in 2 batches.) Mix together the oil, thyme and some salt and pepper and brush over the aubergines. Grill under a preheated medium-hot grill until lightly browned all over, turning once.

3 Beat the ricotta in a bowl with the basil, garlic and a little salt and pepper. Thoroughly drain the pasta sheets and lay them on the work surface. Cut each one in half. Spread the ricotta mixture over the sheets, right to the edges. Arrange the aubergine slices on top. Roll up each pasta sheet to enclose the filling inside.

4 Spread two-thirds of the tomato sauce in a shallow ovenproof dish and arrange the cannelloni on top. Spoon over the remaining tomato sauce and then sprinkle with the cheese. Bake in a preheated oven, 190°C (375°F), Gas Mark 5, for 20 minutes or until the cheese is golden.

4 sheets of fresh or dried lasagne, each about 18 x 15 cm (7 x 6 inches)
2 medium aubergines, thinly sliced
4 tablespoons olive oil
1 teaspoon finely chopped thyme
250 g (8 oz) ricotta cheese
25 g (1 oz) basil leaves, torn into pieces
2 garlic cloves, crushed
1 quantity Fresh Tomato Sauce (see page 249)
100 g (3½ oz) fontina or Gruyère cheese, grated
salt and pepper

Serves **4**
Prep time **30 minutes**
Cooking time **50 minutes**

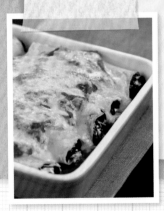

SPAGHETTI CARBONARA

IT'S THE HEAT FROM THE STEAMING HOT SPAGHETTI THAT LIGHTLY COOKS THE CREAMY EGG SAUCE IN THIS RECIPE. THIS IS A QUICKLY ASSEMBLED DISH (MAKE SURE YOU HAVE EVERYTHING READY BEFORE YOU BEGIN).

1 Beat together the egg yolks, whole eggs, cream, Parmesan and plenty of pepper.

2 Heat the oil in a large frying pan and fry the pancetta or bacon for 3-4 minutes or until golden and turning crisp. Add the garlic and cook for a further 1 minute.

3 Meanwhile, bring a large saucepan of lightly salted water to the boil, add the spaghetti and cook for 2 minutes or until tender.

4 Drain the spaghetti and immediately tip it into the frying pan. Turn off the heat and stir in the egg mixture until the eggs are lightly cooked. Serve immediately. (If the heat of the pasta doesn't quite cook the egg sauce, turn on the heat and cook gently and briefly, stirring.)

4 egg yolks
2 eggs
150 ml (¼ pint) single cream
50 g (2 oz) Parmesan cheese, grated
2 tablespoons olive oil
100 g (3½ oz) pancetta or streaky bacon, thinly sliced
2 garlic cloves, crushed
400 g (13 oz) fresh spaghetti
salt and pepper

Serves **4**
Prep time **10 minutes**
Cooking time **5 minutes**

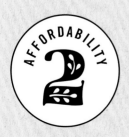

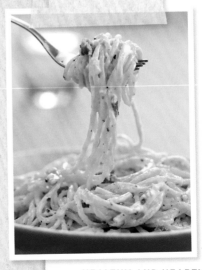

LINGUINE
WITH SHREDDED HAM & EGGS

1 Bring a large saucepan of lightly salted water to the boil to cook the pasta. Meanwhile, mix together the parsley, mustard, lemon juice, sugar, oil and a little salt and pepper. Roll up the ham and slice it as thinly as possible. Trim the spring onions, cut them lengthways into thin shreds, then cut into 5 cm (2 inch) lengths.

2 Put the eggs in a small saucepan and just cover with cold water. Bring to the boil and cook for 4 minutes.

3 Add the pasta to the large saucepan of boiling water, return to the boil and cook for 6-8 minutes or until just tender. Add the spring onions and cook for a further 30 seconds.

4 Drain the pasta and return to the pan. Stir in the ham and the mustard dressing and then pile on to serving plates. Shell and halve the eggs and serve on top.

VARIATION
This recipe is conveniently adaptable. Use other shredded, cooked meats instead of the ham, such as chicken, turkey or pork, if you prefer.

125 g (4 oz) dried linguine
3 tablespoons chopped flat leaf parsley
1 tablespoon wholegrain mustard
2 teaspoons lemon juice
good pinch of caster sugar
3 tablespoons olive oil
100 g (3½ oz) thinly sliced ham
2 spring onions
2 eggs
salt and pepper

Serves **2**
Prep time **5 minutes**
Cooking time **10 minutes**

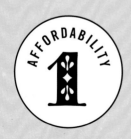

AFFORDABILITY
1

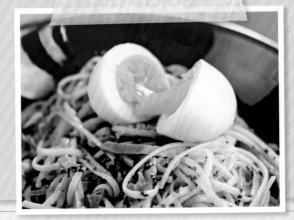

BOLOGNESE SAUCE

BOLOGNESE, OR RAGU, IS USUALLY SERVED WITH TAGLIATELLE. IT SHOULD BE THICK AND PULPY SO IT CLINGS TO THE PASTA IT'S SERVED WITH. IN ITALY, A BOLOGNESE SAUCE IS TOSSED WITH THE PASTA RATHER THAN SPOONED ON TOP.

1 Melt the butter with the oil in a large, heavy-based saucepan and gently fry the onion for 5 minutes. Add the celery and carrot and fry gently for a further 2 minutes.

2 Stir in the garlic, then add the minced beef. Fry gently, breaking up the meat, until lightly browned.

3 Add the wine and let the mixture bubble until the wine reduces slightly. Stir in the chopped tomatoes, tomato paste, oregano and bay leaves and bring to the boil.

4 Reduce the heat and cook very gently, uncovered, for about 45 minutes, stirring occasionally, until the sauce is very thick and pulpy. Remove the bay leaves. Check and adjust the seasoning, then serve with grated Parmesan, if liked.

15 g (½ oz) butter
3 tablespoons olive oil
1 large onion, finely chopped
1 celery stick, finely chopped
1 carrot, finely chopped
3 garlic cloves, crushed
500 g (1 lb) lean minced beef
150 ml (¼ pint) red wine
2 x 400 g (13 oz) cans chopped tomatoes
2 tablespoons sun-dried tomato paste
3 tablespoons chopped oregano
3 bay leaves
salt and pepper
grated Parmesan cheese, to serve (optional)

Serves **4**
Prep time **15 minutes**
Cooking time **1 hour**

AFFORDABILITY **2**

HEALTHY TIP

GET SAUCY Shop-bought sauces can be expensive and many contain more sugar per portion than a builder's first brew of the day. For the cost of a few cans of chopped tomatoes and some garlic and herbs, you can cook up a batch of sauce that's healthier and a whole lot cheaper.

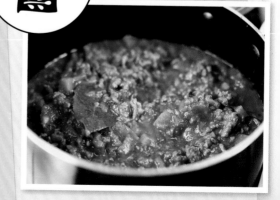

TUNA LAYERED LASAGNE

1 Cook the pasta sheets, in batches, in a large saucepan of lightly salted boiling water according to the packet instructions until al dente. Drain and return to the pan to keep warm.

2 Meanwhile, heat the oil in a frying pan over a medium heat, add the spring onions and courgettes and cook, stirring, for 3 minutes. Remove the pan from the heat, add the tomatoes, tuna and rocket and gently toss everything together.

3 Place a little of the tuna mixture on 4 serving plates and top each portion with a pasta sheet. Spoon over the remaining tuna mixture, then top with the remaining pasta sheets. Season with plenty of pepper and top each with a spoonful of pesto and some basil leaves before serving.

VARIATION

For salmon lasagne, use 400 g (14 oz) fresh salmon fillets. Pan-fry the fillets for 2-3 minutes on each side or until they are cooked through. Remove the bones and skin, then flake the fish and use in place of the tuna.

8 dried lasagne sheets
1 tablespoon olive oil
bunch of spring onions, sliced
2 courgettes, diced
500 g (1 lb) cherry tomatoes, quartered
2 x 200 g (7 oz) cans tuna in water, drained
65 g (2½ oz) rocket
4 teaspoons Pesto (see page 248)
salt and pepper
basil leaves, to garnish

Serves **4**
Prep time **10 minutes**
Cooking time **10 minutes**

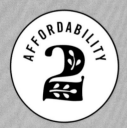

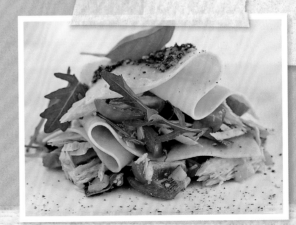

TUNA & OLIVE PASTA

1 Heat the oil in a large frying pan or saucepan and cook the onion over a medium heat for 6-7 minutes until it begins to soften. Add the garlic and cook for a further 1 minute. Pour the chopped tomatoes into the pan with the chilli flakes, if using. Simmer gently for 8-10 minutes, stirring occasionally, until thickened slightly.

2 Meanwhile, bring a large saucepan of lightly salted water to the boil and cook the pasta for 10-12 minutes or according to the packet instructions until just tender. Drain and return to the pan. Stir the tomato sauce into the pasta with the tuna and olives and then heap into 4 dishes to serve.

3 tablespoons olive or vegetable oil
1 red onion, sliced
2 garlic cloves, chopped
2 x 400 g (13 oz) cans chopped tomatoes
½ teaspoon dried chilli flakes (optional)
400 g (13 oz) pasta shapes, such as penne
185 g (6½ oz) can tuna in water or oil, drained and flaked
75 g (3 oz) pitted black or green olives, drained and roughly chopped
salt

Serves **4**
Prep time **10 minutes**
Cooking time **20 minutes**

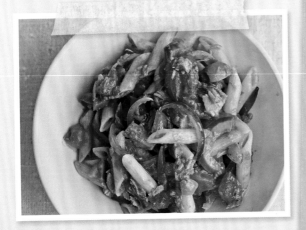

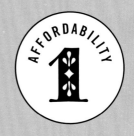
AFFORDABILITY

Salmon
WITH GREEN VEGETABLES

1 Heat the oil in a large, heavy-based frying pan and cook the leek over a medium heat, stirring frequently, for 3 minutes until softened. Add the stock, then bring to the boil and continue boiling for 2 minutes until reduced a little. Add the crème fraîche and stir well to mix. Add the peas, edamame (soya) or broad beans and salmon and return to the boil.

2 Reduce the heat, cover and simmer for 10 minutes until the fish is opaque and cooked through and the peas and beans are piping hot.

3 Sprinkle over the chives and serve spooned over creamy mash with a good grinding of pepper.

1 tablespoon olive oil
1 leek, trimmed, cleaned and thinly sliced
275 ml (9 fl oz) fish stock
200 ml (7 fl oz) half-fat crème fraîche
125 g (4 oz) frozen peas
125 g (4 oz) frozen edamame (soya) or broad beans
4 chunky skinless salmon fillets, about 150 g (5 oz) each
2 tablespoons snipped chives

To serve
mashed potato
pepper

Serves **4**
Prep time **10 minutes**
Cooking time **15 minutes**

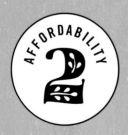

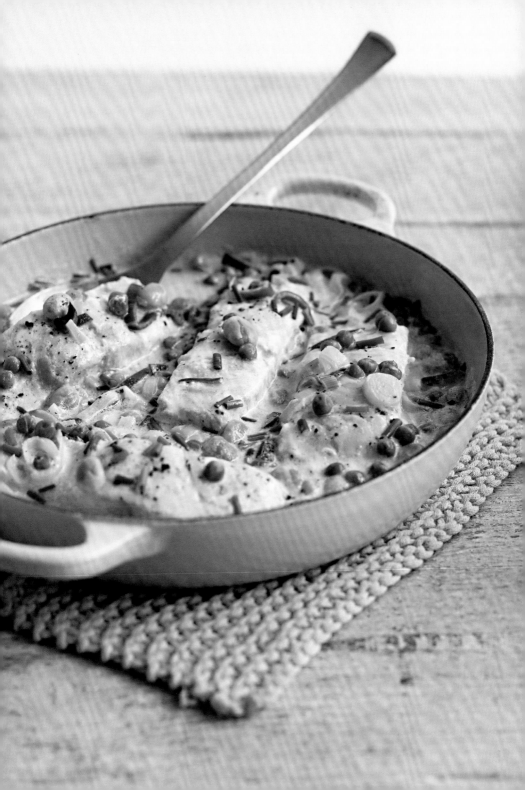

TUNA & JALAPEÑO BAKED POTATOES

1. Prick the potatoes all over with the tip of a sharp knife and place directly in a preheated oven, 180°C (350°F), Gas Mark 4, for 1 hour or until crisp on the outside and the inside is tender. Leave until cool enough to handle.

2. Cut the potatoes in half and scoop the cooked flesh into a bowl. Place the empty potato skins, cut side up, on a baking sheet. Mix the tuna, jalapeño peppers, spring onions, tomatoes and chives into the potato in the bowl. Gently fold in the soured cream, then season to taste with salt and pepper.

3. Spoon the filling into the potato skins, sprinkle with the cheese and cook under a preheated medium-hot grill for 4–5 minutes or until hot and the cheese has melted. Serve immediately with a frisée salad.

VARIATION

For spicy tuna wraps, spoon 4 tablespoons chunky spicy tomato salsa on to 4 large, wholemeal soft flour tortillas. Scatter with the tuna, jalapeño peppers and spring onions. Omit the tomatoes, chives and cheese and top with ½ shredded iceberg lettuce. Roll up the wraps tightly and cut in half diagonally. Serve with a little soured cream, if liked.

4 large baking potatoes
2 x 160 g (5½ oz) cans tuna in spring water, drained
2 tablespoons drained and chopped green jalapeño peppers in brine
2 spring onions, finely chopped
4 firm ripe tomatoes, deseeded and chopped
2 tablespoons snipped chives
3 tablespoons low-fat soured cream
100 g (3½ oz) reduced-fat extra mature Cheddar-style cheese, grated
salt and pepper
frisée salad, to serve

Serves **4**
Prep time **10 minutes, plus cooling**
Cooking time **1 hour 5 minutes**

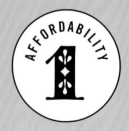

AFFORDABILITY
1

MACARONI CHEESE
SURPRISE

1 Cook the macaroni in a large saucepan of lightly salted boiling water according to the packet instructions until just tender, then drain.

2 Meanwhile, lightly steam all the vegetables over a separate saucepan of boiling water so that they remain crunchy. Drain well.

3 Mix the cornflour and a little of the milk together in a saucepan. Blend to a smooth paste. Add the rest of the milk, then heat gently, whisking continuously until the sauce boils and thickens. Add three-quarters of the cheese, the mustard and cayenne pepper to taste.

4 Mix together the pasta, vegetables and sauce and spoon into an ovenproof dish. Scatter with the remaining cheese and sprinkle with a little cayenne pepper to garnish. Bake in a preheated oven, 200°C (400°F), Gas Mark 6, for about 25 minutes, until golden brown.

VARIATION
Try adding any vegetables, lightly cooked, to the cheesy mixture, such as peas, sweetcorn, mixed peppers, carrots, mushrooms and mixed vegetables.

175 g (6 oz) wholemeal macaroni
2 carrots, cut into small, chunky batons
250 g (8 oz) broccoli florets
1 large leek, trimmed, cleaned and thickly sliced
50 g (2 oz) cornflour
600 ml (1 pint) skimmed milk
100 g (3½ oz) reduced-fat mature Cheddar-style cheese, grated
1 teaspoon mustard
pinch of cayenne pepper, plus extra to garnish
salt

Serves **4**
Prep time **15 minutes**
Cooking time **40 minutes**

HEALTHY TIP

All pasta is naturally healthy – rich in carbohydrates and low in fat. Wholemeal pasta is made from the whole grain and contains more insoluble fibre than the white variety. This type of fibre helps to prevent constipation and other bowel problems.

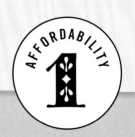

White Bean Gnocchi
WITH SPINACH & PINE NUTS

1 Tip the drained beans into a bowl, then mash with a potato masher or a fork. Beat in the garlic, flour, rosemary and a little salt and pepper. Mix to a thick paste and then turn out on to the work surface. Divide the mixture in half and roll out each piece into a 35 cm (14 inch) sausage. Cut across into 2 cm (¾ inch) pieces.

2 Bring a large saucepan of lightly salted water to the boil. Add the bean gnocchi and cook for 2–3 minutes until the pieces rise to the surface. Remove with a slotted spoon and drain.

3 Heat the oil in a frying pan and fry the pine nuts, stirring until lightly browned. Stir in the water and then add the spinach. Heat gently, turning the spinach in the juices until just beginning to wilt.

4 Dot the cheese into the pan and add the gnocchi. Heat through gently, stirring until the cheese has started to melt. Serve immediately.

400 g (13 oz) can cannellini beans, rinsed and thoroughly drained
1 garlic clove, crushed
50 g (2 oz) plain flour
1 teaspoon finely chopped rosemary
1 tablespoon olive oil
25 g (1 oz) pine nuts
3 tablespoons water
300 g (10 oz) spinach
50 g (2 oz) Gorgonzola cheese
salt and pepper

Serves **2**
Prep time **20 minutes**
Cooking time **8 minutes**

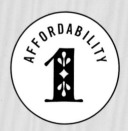

AFFORDABILITY 1

GNOCCHI VERDE

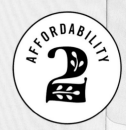

THIS TYPE OF GNOCCHI, SOMETIMES KNOWN AS ROMAN GNOCCHI, USES A SEMOLINA BASE RATHER THAN THE MORE FAMILIAR POTATO. IT'S SOFT AND CREAMY COMFORT FOOD!

1 Grease a 30 x 23 cm (12 x 9 inch) or similar-sized baking dish with butter and line with nonstick baking paper.

2 Put the milk in a large saucepan and bring to the boil. When the milk starts to boil, lower the heat and sprinkle in the semolina flour, in a steady stream, whisking well until the mixture is very thick. Continue beating until the mixture is almost too thick to beat and starts to come away from the sides of the pan.

3 Remove the pan from the heat and dot with 25 g (1 oz) of the butter, add half of the cheese and then the egg yolks. Season with salt and pepper and beat until combined. Turn the mixture into the prepared tin and spread in an even layer with the back of a spoon or palette knife. Leave for at least 30 minutes until cool and set.

4 Put the spinach in the cleaned pan with the water and a generous sprinkling of nutmeg. Cover and cook briefly until the spinach has wilted. Drain well, squeezing out any excess water.

5 Use a 5 cm (2 inch) round cutter to cut the gnocchi into rounds. Chop the trimmings and scatter them in a shallow, 2 litre (3½ pint) ovenproof dish. Spoon the spinach on top. Arrange the gnocchi rounds, slightly overlapping, on top.

6 Melt the remaining butter in a frying pan and fry the shallots until softened. Stir in the cream and spoon over the gnocchi. Scatter with the remaining cheese and bake in a preheated oven, 200°C (400°F), Gas Mark 6, for 20 minutes until pale golden.

75 g (3 oz) butter, plus extra for greasing
1 litre (1¾ pints) milk
200 g (7 oz) semolina flour
100 g (3½ oz) Parmesan-style cheese, grated
3 egg yolks
350 g (11½ oz) spinach
1 tablespoon water
plenty of freshly grated nutmeg
2 shallots, finely chopped
150 ml (¼ pint) single cream
salt and pepper

Serves **4**
Prep time **50 minutes, plus cooling**
Cooking time **30 minutes**

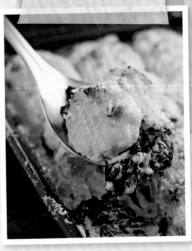

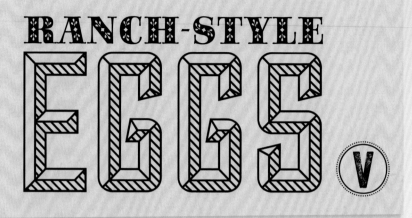

RANCH-STYLE EGGS

V

1 Heat the oil in a large frying pan and add the onion, chilli, garlic, cumin and oregano. Fry gently for about 5 minutes or until soft, then add the tomatoes and peppers and cook for a further 5 minutes. If the sauce looks dry, add a splash of water.

2 Season well with salt and pepper, then make 4 hollows in the mixture, break an egg into each and cover the pan. Cook for 5 minutes or until the eggs are just set.

3 Serve immediately, garnished with chopped coriander.

2 tablespoons olive oil
1 onion, thinly sliced
1 red chilli, deseeded and finely chopped
1 garlic clove, crushed
1 teaspoon ground cumin
1 teaspoon dried oregano
400 g (13 oz) can cherry tomatoes
200 g (7 oz) roasted red and yellow peppers in oil (from a jar), drained and roughly chopped
4 eggs
salt and pepper
4 tablespoons finely chopped fresh coriander, to garnish

Serves **4**
Prep time **10 minutes**
Cooking time **15 minutes**

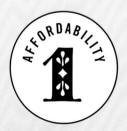

AFFORDABILITY
1

SPINACH & BUTTERNUT LASAGNE

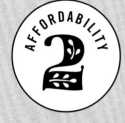

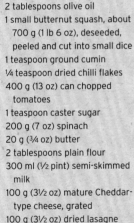

AFFORDABILITY

2 tablespoons olive oil
1 small butternut squash, about
   700 g (1 lb 6 oz), deseeded,
   peeled and cut into small dice
1 teaspoon ground cumin
¼ teaspoon dried chilli flakes
400 g (13 oz) can chopped
   tomatoes
1 teaspoon caster sugar
200 g (7 oz) spinach
20 g (¾ oz) butter
2 tablespoons plain flour
300 ml (½ pint) semi-skimmed
   milk
100 g (3½ oz) mature Cheddar-
   type cheese, grated
100 g (3½ oz) dried lasagne
   sheets
salt and pepper
green salad, to serve

Serves **4**
Prep time **25 minutes**
Cooking time **40 minutes**

1 Heat the oil in a saucepan and gently fry the squash for
5 minutes, stirring. Add the cumin, chilli flakes, tomatoes
and sugar and simmer gently, uncovered, for 20 minutes,
stirring occasionally until the squash is tender. Stir in the
spinach until wilted and season to taste with salt and
pepper. Remove from the heat.

2 Melt the butter in a separate saucepan and stir in the flour,
beating with a wooden spoon for 1 minute. Gradually stir in
the milk and cook over a gentle heat, stirring continuously
until thickened and smooth. Beat in half of the cheese and
season to taste with salt and pepper. Remove from the heat.

3 Spread a quarter of the squash mixture into a shallow,
ovenproof dish and cover with a layer of the lasagne sheets,
breaking them to fit if necessary. Add another quarter of the
squash mixture, spoon over about a third of the cheese
sauce and cover with another layer of the lasagne sheets.
Continue layering the ingredients in the same way, finishing
with a layer of squash mixture topped with cheese sauce.
Sprinkle with the remaining grated cheese.

4 Bake in a preheated oven, 190°C (375°F), Gas Mark 5,
for 40 minutes until golden and bubbling. Serve with a
green salad.

SPINACH & POTATO
TORTILLA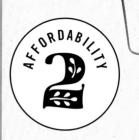

1. Heat the oil in a nonstick, ovenproof frying pan and add the onions and potatoes. Cook over a medium heat for 3-4 minutes or until the vegetables have softened but not coloured, turning and stirring often. Add the garlic, spinach and peppers and stir to mix well.

2. Beat the eggs lightly in a jug and season well with salt and pepper. Pour the eggs into the frying pan, shaking the pan so that the egg mixture is evenly spread. Cook gently for 8-10 minutes or until the tortilla is set at the bottom.

3. Sprinkle over the grated cheese. Place the frying pan under a preheated medium-hot grill and cook for 3-4 minutes or until the top is set and golden.

4. Remove from the heat, cut into 4 wedges and serve warm or at room temperature.

3 tablespoons olive oil
2 onions, finely chopped
250 g (8 oz) cooked potatoes, peeled and cut into 1 cm (½ inch) cubes
2 garlic cloves, finely chopped
200 g (7 oz) cooked spinach, drained thoroughly and roughly chopped
4 tablespoons finely chopped (drained) roasted red peppers (in oil, from a jar)
5 eggs
3-4 tablespoons grated Manchego-style cheese
salt and pepper

Serves **4**
Prep time **10 minutes**
Cooking time **20 minutes**

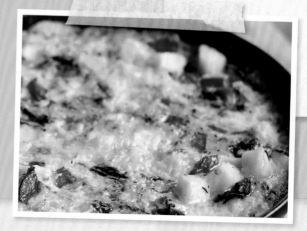

BUTTERNUT SQUASH & RICOTTA FRITTATA

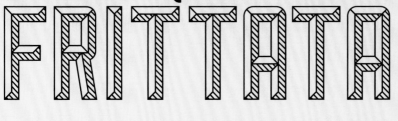

1 Heat the oil in a large, deep, ovenproof frying pan over a medium-low heat, add the onion and butternut squash, then cover loosely and cook gently, stirring frequently, for 18-20 minutes or until softened and golden.

2 Lightly beat the eggs, thyme, sage and ricotta together in a jug, season well with salt and pepper and then pour evenly over the butternut squash. Cook for a further 2-3 minutes until the egg mixture is almost set, stirring occasionally with a heat-resistant rubber spatula to prevent the base from burning.

3 Slide the pan under a preheated medium-hot grill and grill for 3-4 minutes or until the top is set and the frittata is golden. Slice into 6 wedges and serve hot.

1 tablespoon rapeseed oil
1 red onion, thinly sliced
450 g (14½ oz) peeled and deseeded butternut squash, diced
8 eggs
1 tablespoon chopped thyme
2 tablespoons chopped sage
125 g (4 oz) ricotta cheese
salt and pepper

Serves **6**
Prep time **10 minutes**
Cooking time **25-30 minutes**

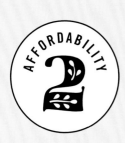

AFFORDABILITY
2

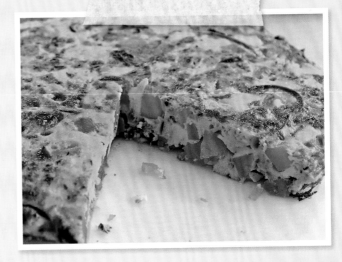

BRAIN FOOD

You'll need all the brain capacity you can muster while you're studying, so it makes sense to ensure your diet includes foods that can help you reach your maximum potential. Certain foods contain essential nutrients that will help you concentrate and focus when you're studying and revising, and help to naturally calm your nerves and stop you stressing out before exams.

BRIGHT MEAL IDEAS

BREAKFAST
Yogurt The probiotics in live yogurt, along with the calcium, make it the perfect choice for the first meal of the day. Spoon over your granola or cereal and top with a drizzle of honey.

Marmite Love it or loathe it, with its vitamin B and iron content this should be the spread of choice for your morning toast.

LUNCH
Wholegrain bread Slow-release carbohydrates are needed at lunchtime to keep you feeling full and able to concentrate throughout the afternoon.

Eggs Protein should be present at every meal and if you combine your wholegrain bread with an egg filling, you've got it covered. Eggs could help to improve your cognitive skills, which makes them the perfect student food.

DINNER
Salmon Omega-3-rich salmon is the ideal choice for a healthy supper as it can contribute to healthy brain function. Choose fresh salmon steaks or fillets, or try adding smoked salmon to pasta dishes.

Broccoli Team your salmon with a heap of steamed broccoli and you'll be the brightest student in the lecture hall.

BRAINY SNACKS
Nuts and seeds These handy snacks are a really good source of vitamin E.

Bananas With potassium and serotonin-producing tryptophan, these provide the ideal snack for focusing on the task in hand. Bananas are also believed to aid sleep, so if you need to wind down after studying, peel and chomp one before bedtime.

Dark chocolate If you need an excuse to nibble on a square or two of dark chocolate, then remind yourself that it can aid blood flow to the brain… and keep nibbling.

SUPERFOODS

There's much debate about whether certain foods should be singled out for being 'superfoods'. But there's no denying that these ingredients could give you a boost in the brain cell department.

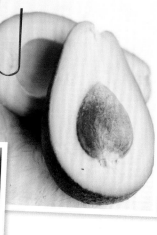

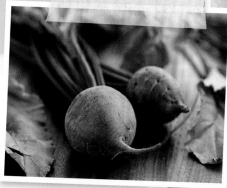

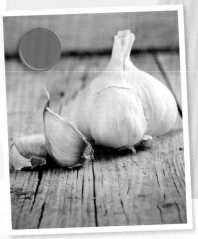

Pumpkin seeds
Blueberries
Green tea

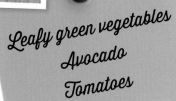

Leafy green vegetables
Avocado
Tomatoes

Garlic
Beetroot

KEDGEREE-STYLE RICE
WITH SPINACH

1 Place the haddock and peas in a frying pan, cover with the boiling water and bring to the boil. Reduce the heat, cover and simmer for 3-4 minutes, adding the spinach for the final minute of cooking.

2 Meanwhile, microwave the express rice for 5 minutes or according to the packet instructions. Drain the fish, spinach and peas and flake the fish. Return to the pan and add the butter, garam masala and rice, season with pepper and toss well. Serve sprinkled with parsley, if liked.

250 g (8 oz) smoked haddock fillets
125 g (4 oz) frozen peas
150 ml (¼ pint) boiling water
250 g (8 oz) spinach leaves
500 g (1 lb) express rice
25 g (1 oz) butter
½ teaspoon garam masala
pepper
3 tablespoons chopped parsley, to garnish (optional)

Serves **4**
Prep time **5 minutes**
Cooking time **5 minutes**

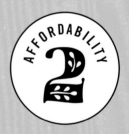

AFFORDABILITY

2

BARLEY & GINGER
RISOTTO
WITH BUTTERNUT SQUASH

1 Cut the squash into 2 cm (¾ inch) cubes, discarding the skin and any seeds. Put in an ovenproof casserole with the onion and oil and stir to mix. Bake, covered, in a preheated oven 180°C (350°F), Gas Mark 4, for 30 minutes.

2 Stir in the garlic, pearl barley, rosemary, ginger and stock. Return to the oven, uncovered, and bake for a further 50 minutes. Stir the risotto occasionally during cooking until the barley is tender, adding a little more water if the consistency runs dry.

3 Remove the rosemary stalks. Season the risotto with plenty of pepper and stir in the soured cream. Spoon into bowls and serve sprinkled with cheese, if liked.

600 g (1 lb 2 oz) butternut squash
1 onion, chopped
1 tablespoon olive or sunflower oil
2 garlic cloves, thinly sliced
150 g (5 oz) pearl barley
2 large sprigs of rosemary
2 cm (¾ inch) piece of fresh root
  ginger, peeled and chopped
300 ml (½ pint) Vegetable Stock
  (see page 244)
4 tablespoons low-fat soured
  cream
pepper
grated Parmesan-style cheese,
  to serve (optional)

Serves **2**
Prep time **15 minutes**
Cooking time **1 hour 20 minutes**

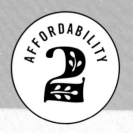

LEMON & HERB RISOTTO

1 Heat the oil in a heavy-based saucepan and add the shallots, garlic, celery, courgette and carrot and fry gently for 4 minutes or until the vegetables have softened. Add the rice and turn up the heat. Stir-fry for 2-3 minutes.

2 Add a ladleful of hot stock followed by half of the herbs and season well with salt and pepper. Reduce the heat to medium-low and add the remaining stock, 1 ladleful at a time, stirring constantly until each amount is absorbed and the rice is just firm to the bite but cooked through.

3 Remove from the heat and gently stir in the remaining herbs, the butter, lemon rind and cheese. Place the lid on the pan and allow to sit for 2-3 minutes, during which time it will become creamy and oozy. Serve immediately, sprinkled with pepper.

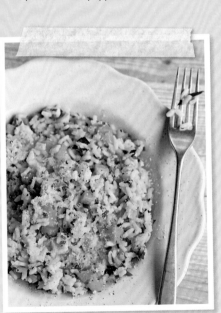

1 tablespoon olive oil
3 shallots, finely chopped
2 cloves garlic, finely chopped
1 head of celery, finely chopped
1 courgette, finely diced
1 carrot, finely diced
300 g (10 oz) arborio rice
1.2 litres (2 pints) hot Vegetable Stock (see page 244)
good handful of fresh mixed herbs, such as tarragon, parsley, chives and dill
100 g (3½ oz) butter
1 tablespoon finely grated lemon rind
100 g (3½ oz) Parmesan-style cheese, grated
salt and pepper

Serves **4**
Prep time **10 minutes**
Cooking time **30 minutes, plus standing**

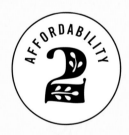

MIXED BEAN & TOMATO
CHILLI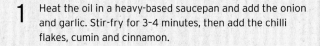

1 Heat the oil in a heavy-based saucepan and add the onion and garlic. Stir-fry for 3-4 minutes, then add the chilli flakes, cumin and cinnamon.

2 Stir-fry for 2-3 minutes, then stir in the tomatoes. Bring to the boil, reduce the heat to medium and simmer gently for 10 minutes.

3 Stir in all the beans (and chilli sauce) and cook for 3-4 minutes until warmed through. Season well with salt and pepper and ladle into 4 bowls to serve.

4 Top each serving with a tablespoon of soured cream, garnish with chopped coriander and serve immediately with corn tortillas.

2 tablespoons olive oil
1 onion, finely chopped
4 garlic cloves, crushed
1 teaspoon dried chilli flakes
2 teaspoons ground cumin
1 teaspoon ground cinnamon
400 g (13 oz) can chopped
    tomatoes
400 g (13 oz) can mixed beans,
    rinsed and drained
400 g (13 oz) can red kidney beans
    in chilli sauce
salt and pepper

To serve
4 tablespoons low-fat soured
    cream
25 g (1 oz) finely chopped fresh
    coriander, to garnish
warmed corn tortillas

Serves **4**
Prep time **10 minutes**
Cooking time **25 minutes**

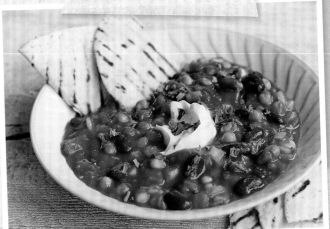

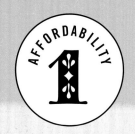

AFFORDABILITY
1

CAULIFLOWER & CHICKPEA CURRY (V)

1 Heat the oil in a large, nonstick frying pan over a medium heat. Add the spring onions and stir-fry for 2-3 minutes. Add the garlic, ginger and curry powder and stir-fry for 20-30 seconds until fragrant. Add the cauliflower and peppers and stir-fry for a further 2-3 minutes.

2 Stir in the tomatoes and bring to the boil. Cover, reduce the heat a little and simmer for 10 minutes, stirring occasionally. Add the chickpeas, season to taste with salt and pepper and bring back to the boil.

3 Remove from the heat and serve immediately with steamed rice and mint raita, if liked.

VARIATION
For broccoli and black-eye bean curry, follow the recipe above, replacing the cauliflower with 300 g (10 oz) broccoli florets and the chickpeas with a 400 g (13 oz) can black-eye beans.

AFFORDABILITY
1

1 tablespoon groundnut oil
8 spring onions, cut into 5 cm (2 inch) lengths
2 teaspoons grated garlic
2 teaspoons ground ginger
2 tablespoons medium curry powder
300 g (10 oz) cauliflower florets
1 red pepper, cored, deseeded and diced
1 yellow pepper, cored, deseeded and diced
400 g (13 oz) can chopped tomatoes
400 g (13 oz) can chickpeas, rinsed and drained
salt and pepper

To serve
Boiled Rice (see page 247) (optional)
mint raita (optional)

Serves **4**
Prep time **10 minutes**
Cooking time **20 minutes**

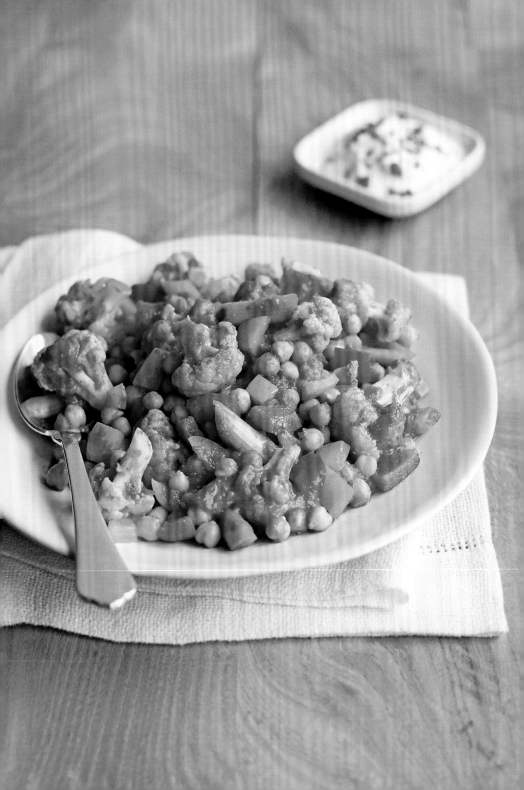

VEGETABLE CURRY WITH RICE

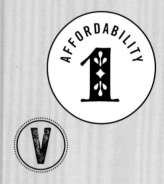

1 Heat the oil in a large frying pan and cook the onion and mixed vegetables over a medium heat for about 10 minutes, stirring frequently, until lightly coloured and beginning to soften. Stir in the garlic and ginger and cook for a further 2 minutes, then add the curry paste and stir over the heat for 1 minute to cook the spices.

2 Pour in the chopped tomatoes and stock, then bring to the boil, reduce the heat and simmer gently for about 15 minutes, stirring occasionally, until the curry has thickened slightly and the vegetables are tender. Serve spooned over boiled rice.

2 tablespoons vegetable oil
1 onion, roughly chopped
600 g (1 lb 2 oz) mixed chopped vegetables, such as carrots, leeks, swede, potato, cauliflower and broccoli
2 garlic cloves, chopped
2.5 cm (1 inch) piece of fresh root ginger, peeled and chopped
4 tablespoons medium-hot curry paste, such as rogan josh or balti
400 g (13 oz) can chopped tomatoes
400 ml (14 fl oz) Vegetable Stock (see page 244)
Boiled Rice (see page 247), to serve

Serves **4**
Prep time **10 minutes**
Cooking time **30 minutes**

Vegetable, Fruit & Nut BIRYANI

1. Bring a large saucepan of lightly salted water to the boil and cook the rice for 5 minutes. Add the cauliflower and cook with the rice for a further 10 minutes or until both are tender, then drain.

2. Meanwhile, heat the oil in a large, heavy-based frying pan and cook the sweet potatoes and onion over a medium heat, stirring occasionally, for 10 minutes until browned and tender. Add the curry paste, turmeric and mustard seeds and cook, stirring, for a further 2 minutes.

3. Pour in the stock and add the green beans. Bring to the boil, then reduce the heat and simmer for 5 minutes. Stir in the drained rice and cauliflower, the sultanas, coriander and cashew nuts and simmer for a further 2 minutes. Spoon on to serving plates and serve with poppadums and raita.

250 g (8 oz) basmati rice
½ cauliflower, broken into florets
2 tablespoons vegetable oil
2 large sweet potatoes, peeled and cut into cubes
1 large onion, sliced
3 tablespoons hot curry paste
½ teaspoon ground turmeric
2 teaspoons mustard seeds
300 ml (½ pint) Vegetable Stock (see page 244)
250 g (8 oz) fine green beans, topped, tailed and cut in half
100 g (3½ oz) sultanas
6 tablespoons chopped fresh coriander
50 g (2 oz) cashew nuts, lightly toasted
salt

To serve
poppadums
raita

Serves **4**
Prep time **10 minutes**
Cooking time **25 minutes**

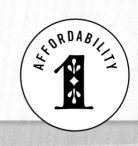

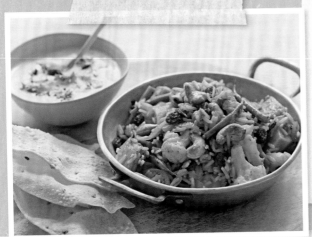

BAKED
SWEET POTATOES

1 Put the potatoes on a baking tray and roast in a preheated oven, 220°C (425°F), Gas Mark 7, for 45-50 minutes until cooked through.

2 Combine the soured cream, spring onions, chives and salt and pepper in a bowl.

3 Cut the baked potatoes in half lengthways, top with the butter and spoon over the soured cream mixture. Serve immediately.

4 sweet potatoes, about 250 g (8 oz) each, scrubbed
200 ml (7 fl oz) low-fat soured cream
2 spring onions, finely chopped
1 tablespoon snipped chives
50 g (2 oz) butter
salt and pepper

Serves **4**
Prep time **5 minutes**
Cooking time **45-50 minutes**

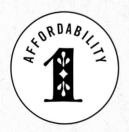

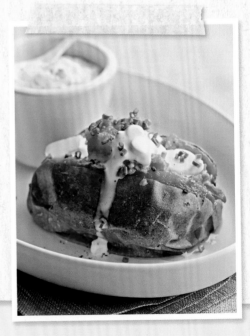

Caribbean Chicken
WITH RICE & PEAS

1 Mix together the jerk seasoning, ginger and lime juice in a non-metallic bowl. Cut a few slashes across each chicken breast and coat in the mixture. Heat 2 tablespoons of the oil in a frying pan, add the chicken and cook over a medium heat for 15–20 minutes, turning occasionally, until cooked through.

2 Meanwhile, heat the remaining oil in a saucepan, add the onion and garlic and cook for 2 minutes until slightly softened. Add the rice, stock and coconut milk and bring to the boil, then reduce the heat, cover and simmer for 15–20 minutes until the liquid has been absorbed and the rice is tender, adding the kidney beans, sweetcorn and thyme sprigs for the final 5 minutes.

3 Slice the chicken and serve with the rice mixture and lime wedges, garnished with a few sprigs of thyme.

2 teaspoons jerk seasoning
1 teaspoon peeled and grated
   fresh root ginger
juice of 1 lime
2 boneless, skinless chicken
   breasts, about 150 g (5 oz) each
3 tablespoons vegetable oil
1 small onion, chopped
1 garlic clove, crushed
150 g (5 oz) long-grain rice
175 ml (6 fl oz) Chicken Stock
   (see page 244)
175 ml (6 fl oz) coconut milk
200 g (7 oz) can red kidney beans,
   rinsed and drained
50 g (2 oz) frozen or canned
   sweetcorn
few thyme sprigs, plus extra
   to garnish
lime wedges, to serve

Serves **2**
Prep time **10 minutes**
Cooking time **25 minutes**

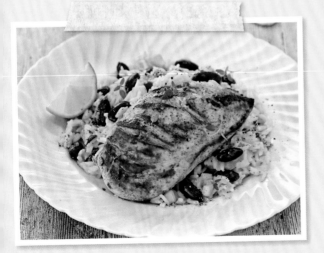

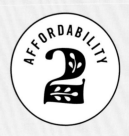

AFFORDABILITY
2

LENTIL & CHICKEN STEW

1 Heat the oil in a medium, heavy-based frying pan and cook the chicken and celery for 5 minutes. Add the fresh tomatoes and stir for 1 minute.

2 Add the lentils, canned tomatoes, stock cube and water. Bring to the boil and boil for 2 minutes, stirring occasionally.

3 Stir in the chopped parsley, then ladle into serving bowls and serve with crusty bread to mop up the juices, if liked.

VARIATION

For a thick red lentil and chicken stew, heat 1 tablespoon olive oil and cook 2 x 150 g (5 oz) thinly sliced chicken breasts, 1 thinly sliced large onion and 4 chopped celery sticks over a medium-high heat for 5 minutes. Add 4 roughly chopped tomatoes, 250 g (8 oz) red lentils, 400 g (13 oz) can chopped tomatoes and 600 ml (1 pint) Chicken Stock (see page 244). Bring to the boil, then reduce the heat, cover and simmer, stirring occasionally, for 20 minutes or until the lentils are soft and tender. Season to taste with salt and pepper and stir in 6 tablespoons chopped parsley. Serve with warm crusty bread.

1 tablespoon olive oil
2 chicken breasts, about 150 g (5 oz) each, thinly sliced
3 celery sticks, roughly chopped
4 tomatoes, roughly chopped
250 g (8 oz) ready-cooked Puy lentils
400 g (13 oz) can chopped tomatoes
1 chicken stock cube, crumbled
150 ml (¼ pint) boiling water
2 tablespoons chopped parsley
crusty bread, to serve (optional)

Serves **4**
Prep time **10 minutes**
Cooking time **10 minutes**

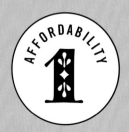

AFFORDABILITY
1

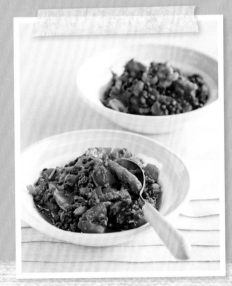

French-style CHICKEN STEW

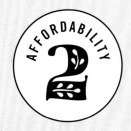

1 Place the leek, chicken, potatoes and carrot in a large saucepan. Pour in the stock and wine and season to taste with salt and pepper. Bring to the boil, then reduce the heat and simmer for 15 minutes, stirring occasionally, until just cooked through.

2 Stir in the peas and crème fraîche and heat through. Scatter over the tarragon and serve immediately.

VARIATION

For a chicken sauté with peas, lettuce and tarragon, heat 1 tablespoon oil in a saucepan. Add 300 g (10 oz) thinly sliced chicken breasts and cook for 2 minutes until golden. Add 1 crushed garlic clove and cook for a further 30 seconds. Pour in 25 ml (1 fl oz) dry white wine and bubble for 1 minute, then add 50 ml (2 fl oz) Chicken Stock (see page 244) and boil hard for 2 minutes. Stir in 100 g (3½ oz) defrosted frozen peas, 1 sliced Little Gem lettuce and 2 tablespoons crème fraîche, season to taste with salt and pepper and heat through. Sprinkle with chopped tarragon and serve with lightly toasted baguette slices.

1 leek, trimmed, cleaned and sliced
4 boneless, skinless chicken thighs, cut into chunks
400 g (13 oz) small new potatoes, halved
1 carrot, sliced
400 ml (14 fl oz) Chicken Stock (see page 244)
50 ml (2 fl oz) dry white wine
100 g (3½ oz) frozen peas, defrosted
2 tablespoons half-fat crème fraîche
salt and pepper
handful of chopped tarragon, to garnish

Serves **4**
Prep time **10 minutes**
Cooking time **20 minutes**

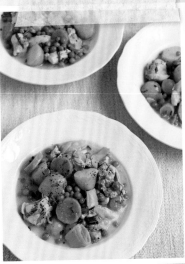

CHICKEN & SPINACH STEW

1 Mix the chicken with the ground spices until well coated. Heat the oil in a large saucepan or flameproof casserole, then add the chicken and cook for 2–3 minutes, until lightly browned.

2 Stir in the tomato purée, tomatoes, raisins, lentils and lemon rind, season with salt and pepper and simmer gently, stirring occasionally, for about 12 minutes, until thickened slightly and the chicken is cooked.

3 Add the spinach and stir until wilted. Ladle the stew into serving bowls, then scatter with the parsley and serve with steamed couscous or rice.

VARIATION

For chicken and rice soup with lemon, heat 2 tablespoons olive oil in a large saucepan and cook 4 sliced spring onions and 2 chopped garlic cloves over a medium heat for 2–3 minutes, to soften. Add 200 g (7 oz) thinly sliced, boneless, skinless chicken breasts and cook for 3–4 minutes, until lightly browned all over. Add 150 g (5 oz) long-grain rice and stir to coat in the oil. Pour 1.2 litres (2 pints) Chicken or Vegetable Stock (see pages 244) into the pan, season to taste with salt and pepper, add a pinch of freshly grated nutmeg, then simmer, covered, for about 15 minutes, until the rice is tender. Stir 150 g (5 oz) mixed chopped watercress and spinach leaves into the soup and stir for 1–2 minutes, until the leaves have wilted. Ladle into bowls and serve with lemon wedges.

625 g (1¼ lb) boneless, skinless chicken thighs, thinly sliced
2 teaspoons ground cumin
1 teaspoon ground ginger
2 tablespoons olive oil
1 tablespoon tomato purée
2 x 400 g (13 oz) cans cherry tomatoes
50 g (2 oz) raisins
250 g (8 oz) ready-cooked Puy lentils
1 teaspoon finely grated lemon rind
150 g (5 oz) baby spinach
salt and pepper
handful of chopped parsley, to garnish
steamed couscous or Boiled Rice (see page 247), to serve

Serves **4**
Prep time **10 minutes**
Cooking time **20 minutes**

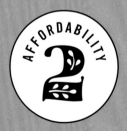

AFFORDABILITY 2

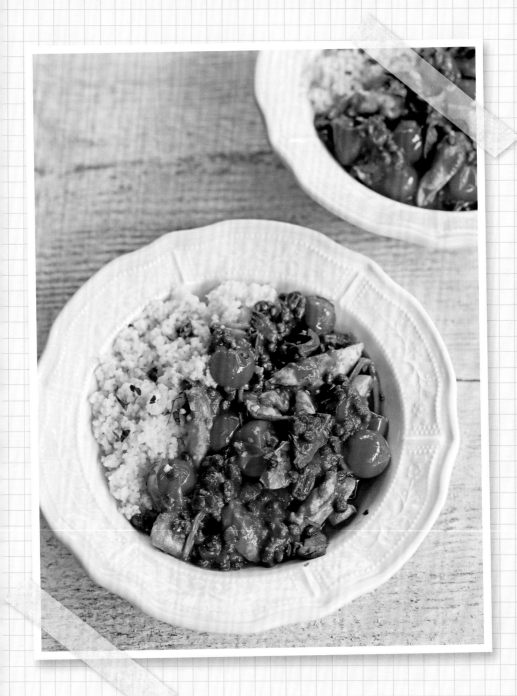

CHICKEN
JALFREZI

1 Heat the oil in a large frying pan, add the chicken, onion and green pepper and cook over a medium heat, stirring occasionally, for 10 minutes until starting to turn golden. Add the chilli and spices and cook for 2–3 minutes, then stir in the tomatoes and cook for a further 3 minutes.

2 Stir in the yogurt, then pour in the water, cover and simmer very gently for 10 minutes until the chicken is cooked through and the flavours have infused, stirring occasionally and adding a little more water if necessary. Serve with warm naan bread to mop up the juices.

2 tablespoons sunflower oil
300 g (10 oz) boneless, skinless chicken breasts, cut into pieces
1 onion, cut into thin wedges
1 small green pepper, cored, deseeded and cut into chunks
1 green chilli, deseeded and finely chopped
1 teaspoon ground cumin
1 teaspoon garam masala
½ teaspoon ground turmeric
2 tomatoes, cut into wedges
2 tablespoons natural yogurt
200 ml (7 fl oz) hot water
warm naan bread, to serve

Serves **2**
Prep time **15 minutes**
Cooking time **30 minutes**

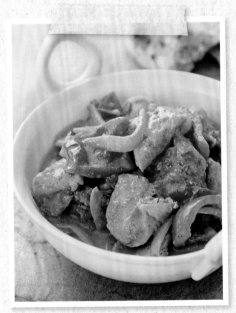

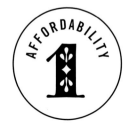

CHICKEN SHAWARMA

1 Heat the oil in a small frying pan and fry the onion for 3 minutes until softened. Add the chicken and fry for a further 5 minutes, stirring frequently until the chicken is cooked through. Stir in the shawarma spice and cook for a further 1 minute.

2 Lightly toast the pitta bread. Mix the tahini with the honey, vinegar and hot water in a small bowl. Season lightly with salt and pepper.

3 Shred the lettuce on a serving plate and pile the chicken mixture on top. Scatter with the gherkin and spoon over the tahini dressing. Serve with the toasted pitta bread.

1 teaspoon olive or vegetable oil
½ onion, thinly sliced
200 g (7 oz) boneless, skinless chicken thighs, cut into large pieces
1 teaspoon shawarma spice
1 wholemeal pitta bread
1 tablespoon tahini
1 teaspoon clear honey
1 teaspoon white or red wine vinegar
4 teaspoons hot water
1 Little Gem lettuce
1 gherkin, sliced
salt and pepper

Serves **1**
Prep time **10 minutes**
Cooking time **10 minutes**

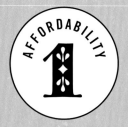

JAMBALAYA
WITH CHORIZO & PEPPERS

1 Cook the rice in a large saucepan of boiling water for about 25 minutes until tender. Drain.

2 Meanwhile, heat the oil in a frying pan and gently fry the onion, peppers and chorizo for 10-15 minutes, stirring occasionally, until softened and beginning to brown.

3 Stir in the tomatoes, allspice and sugar and cook for 5 minutes until the tomato juices are reduced. Stir in the cooked rice and peas and season to taste with salt and pepper. Heat through for 5 minutes, then serve.

150 g (5 oz) brown basmati rice
1 tablespoon olive oil
1 onion, chopped
1 red pepper, cored, deseeded and chopped
1 yellow pepper, cored, deseeded and chopped
150 g (5 oz) spicy chorizo sausage, diced
400 g (13 oz) can chopped tomatoes
¼ teaspoon ground allspice
1 teaspoon caster sugar
100g (3½ oz) frozen peas
salt and pepper

Serves **3**
Prep time **15 minutes**
Cooking time **30 minutes**

HEALTHY TIP

STICK TO USE-BY DATES Food poisoning is a daily danger for students preparing food in less than salubrious surroundings. Lower your chances by sticking to the advice on food labels — if it's use by today don't let it fester in the fridge for another couple of nights.

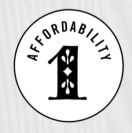

Chicken Burgers
WITH TOMATO SALSA

1 Mix together all the burger ingredients, except the oil. Divide the mixture into 4 and form each portion into a burger. Cover and chill for 30 minutes.

2 Combine all the salsa ingredients in a bowl. Cover and set aside.

3 Brush the burgers with the oil and cook under a preheated high grill or on a preheated barbecue for about 3–4 minutes each side until cooked through. Serve each burger in a bread roll with the tomato salsa and some salad leaves.

VARIATION
For chilli and coriander chicken burgers with mango salsa, make the burgers as above, replacing the sun-dried tomatoes with a finely chopped deseeded red chilli (and using coriander pesto in place of the standard pesto). Serve with a salsa made from 1 peeled and stoned large ripe mango, 1 small red onion and 1 deseeded red chilli, all finely chopped, then mixed with 2 tablespoons chopped fresh coriander, 2 tablespoons chopped mint leaves, juice of 1 lime and 2 teaspoons olive oil.

1 garlic clove, crushed
3 spring onions, thinly sliced
1 tablespoon Pesto (see page 248)
2 tablespoons chopped mixed herbs, such as parsley, tarragon and thyme
375 g (12 oz) minced chicken
2 sun-dried tomatoes, finely chopped
1 teaspoon olive oil

Tomato salsa
250 g (8 oz) cherry tomatoes, quartered
1 red chilli, deseeded and finely chopped
1 tablespoon chopped fresh coriander
finely grated rind and juice of 1 lime

To serve
4 bread rolls
salad leaves

Serves **4**
Prep time **15 minutes, plus chilling**
Cooking time **10 minutes**

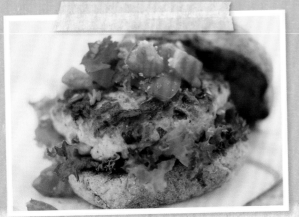

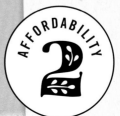

AFFORDABILITY

CHICKEN FAJITAS
WITH NO-CHILLI SALSA

1 To make the chicken fajitas, place all the ground spices, garlic and chopped coriander in a mixing bowl. Cut the chicken into bite-sized strips and toss in the oil, then add to the spices and toss to coat lightly in the spice mixture.

2 Make the salsa. Mix the tomatoes, coriander and cucumber in a bowl and drizzle over the oil. Transfer to a serving bowl.

3 Make the guacamole. Mash the avocado in a bowl with the lime rind and juice and sweet chilli sauce, if using, until soft and rough-textured.

4 Heat a griddle pan or heavy-based frying pan until hot and cook the chicken for 3–4 minutes, turning occasionally, until golden and cooked through. Top the tortillas with the hot chicken strips, guacamole and salsa, and fold into quarters to serve.

VARIATION

For soured cream chicken tacos, cook the chicken as above and spoon into 8 warmed, ready-made taco shells. Serve 2 per person with 1½ teaspoons low-fat soured cream and some fresh coriander leaves on each.

½ teaspoon ground coriander
½ teaspoon ground cumin
½ teaspoon paprika
1 garlic clove, crushed
3 tablespoons chopped fresh
   coriander
375 g (12 oz) boneless, skinless
   chicken breasts
1 tablespoon olive oil
4 soft flour tortillas

Salsa
3 ripe tomatoes, finely chopped
3 tablespoons chopped fresh
   coriander
⅛ cucumber, finely chopped
1 tablespoon olive oil

Guacamole
1 large ripe avocado, peeled,
   stoned and chopped
finely grated rind and juice of
   ½ lime
sweet chilli sauce, to taste
   (optional)

Serves **4**
Prep time **20 minutes**
Cooking time **5 minutes**

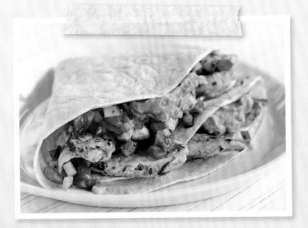

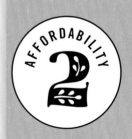

AFFORDABILITY 2

POT ROAST CHICKEN

THIS DISH MAKES A DELIGHTFUL CHANGE FROM A TRADITIONAL ROAST CHICKEN. IF YOU HAVE ANY LEFTOVER CHICKEN, MIX WITH MAYO AND SHREDDED LETTUCE FOR AN EASY SANDWICH FILLING.

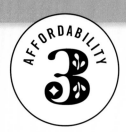

1 Season the chicken all over with salt and pepper. Melt the butter with the oil in a frying pan and fry the chicken on all sides. Transfer to a large, ovenproof casserole.

2 Fry the onion and celery in the pan juices for 6-8 minutes or until browned. Stir in the garlic, wine and herbs and pour over the chicken. Cover and bake in a preheated oven, 160°C (325°F), Gas Mark 3, for 1 hour.

3 Meanwhile, rinse the lentils and put them in a saucepan with plenty of water. Bring to the boil and boil for 10 minutes. Drain well.

4 Tip the lentils around the chicken and return to the oven for a further 45 minutes. Transfer the cooked chicken and lentil mixture to a warmed serving dish and cover. Remember to remove the bay leaves and thyme stalks before serving.

5 Mix the capers, parsley and crème fraîche together in a small pan and heat through gently, stirring. Serve with the carved chicken and the lentil mixture.

1.5 kg (3 lb) oven-ready chicken
25 g (1 oz) butter
2 tablespoons olive oil
1 onion, sliced
3 celery sticks, sliced
4-6 garlic cloves, crushed
250 ml (8 fl oz) dry white wine
3 bay leaves
sprigs of thyme
150 g (5 oz) Puy lentils
2 tablespoons capers, drained
4 tablespoons chopped parsley
100 ml (3½ fl oz) half-fat crème fraîche
salt and pepper

Serves **4**
Prep time **15 minutes**
Cooking time **2 hours**

ROASTED LEMONY CHICKEN WITH COURGETTES

1 Cut a few slashes across each chicken thigh. Mix together the lemon rind, crushed garlic and 2 tablespoons of the oil in a bowl, then rub this mixture over the chicken thighs, pushing it into the slashes.

2 Place the chicken in a roasting tin with the potatoes and season with salt and pepper. Roast in a preheated oven, 220°C (425°F), Gas Mark 7, for 10 minutes.

3 Add the onion, courgette, unpeeled garlic cloves and thyme leaves to the tin and drizzle with the remaining oil. Return to the oven and roast for a further 15 minutes or until the chicken is golden and cooked through and the vegetables are tender.

4 Squeeze the soft garlic over the chicken and vegetables, discarding the skin, and serve garnished with thyme sprigs.

4 chicken thighs, about 100 g
    (3½ oz) each
finely grated rind of 1 lemon
1 garlic clove, crushed, plus
    2 whole cloves, unpeeled
4 tablespoons olive oil
375 g (12 oz) new potatoes,
    halved if large
1 red onion, cut into wedges
1 courgette, thickly sliced
1 tablespoon thyme leaves, plus
    a few sprigs to garnish
salt and pepper

Serves **2**
Prep time **10 minutes**
Cooking time **25 minutes**

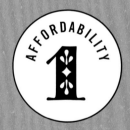

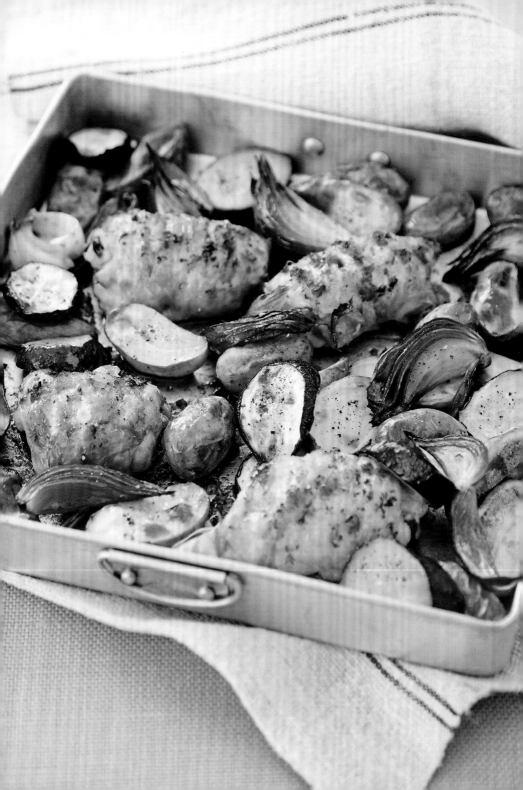

WARM CHICKEN, MED VEG & BULGAR WHEAT SALAD

1. Heat 5 tablespoons of the oil in a large frying pan, add the courgette, onion, red pepper, aubergine and garlic and cook over a high heat for 15-20 minutes, stirring regularly until golden and softened.

2. Meanwhile, cook the bulgar wheat in a saucepan of lightly salted boiling water for 15 minutes until tender.

3. While the bulgar wheat is cooking, brush the remaining oil over the chicken breasts and season well with salt and pepper. Heat a large griddle pan until smoking, then add the chicken and cook over a high heat for 4-5 minutes on each side or until golden and cooked through. Remove from the heat and thinly slice diagonally.

4. Drain the bulgar wheat. Place in a large bowl, toss with the parsley and season with salt and pepper. Add the hot vegetables and chicken, toss together and serve.

6 tablespoons olive oil
1 large courgette, cut into thick slices
1 large red onion, cut into thin wedges
1 red pepper, cored, deseeded and cut into chunks
½ small aubergine, cut into small chunks
1 garlic clove, thinly sliced
150 g (5 oz) bulgar wheat
4 chicken breasts, about 150 g (5 oz) each
4 tablespoons chopped parsley
salt and pepper

Serves **4**
Prep time **15 minutes**
Cooking time **20 minutes**

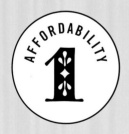

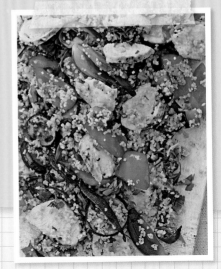

OVEN-BAKED TURKEY & GRUYÈRE BURGERS

1. Thinly slice half of the onion and reserve. Finely chop the remainder and mix in a bowl with the minced turkey, dried herbs and a little salt and pepper. Divide into 4 even-sized portions. Cut the Gruyère into 4 pieces and push a piece into the centre of each portion of minced turkey. Flatten out into burger shapes.

2. Brush a baking sheet with a little of the oil and place the burgers on top. Brush the burgers with the remaining oil, then bake in a preheated oven, 200°C (400°F), Gas Mark 6, for 20 minutes, turning the burgers halfway through cooking.

3. Halve the buns. Stir the walnuts into the mayonnaise and season with pepper. Place the burgers on the bun bases and top with the walnut mayonnaise, watercress and sliced onion. Top with the burger lids and serve.

1 small red onion
500g (1lb) minced turkey
½ teaspoon dried thyme or oregano
90 g (3¼ oz) Gruyère cheese
1 teaspoon olive or sunflower oil
2 seeded buns
25 g (1 oz) walnuts, finely chopped
4 tablespoons mayonnaise
50 g (2 oz) watercress
salt and pepper

Serves **4**
Prep time **10 minutes**
Cooking time **20 minutes**

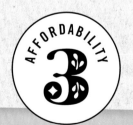

AFFORDABILITY
3

SWEDISH MEATBALLS

COATED IN A SWEET, SPICY CRANBERRY GLAZE, THESE BITE-SIZED MEATBALLS MAKE A GOOD STUDENT SUPPER DISH SERVED WITH PAPPARDELLE OR TAGLIATELLE. MIXING THE MEAT AND FLAVOURINGS IN A BLENDER OR FOOD PROCESSOR GIVES THE MEATBALLS THEIR CHARACTERISTIC SMOOTH TEXTURE.

1 Make the cranberry glaze. Combine the cranberry sauce, stock, chilli sauce and lemon juice in a small saucepan and heat gently until smooth, stirring, then simmer gently for 5 minutes. Remove from the heat and set aside.

2 Meanwhile, put the minced veal and pork in a food processor with the onion, garlic, breadcrumbs, egg yolk, parsley and a little salt and pepper, and process until the mixture forms a fairly smooth paste that clings together.

3 Scoop teaspoonfuls of the paste and roll them into small balls between the palms of your hands.

4 Heat the oil in a large, heavy-based frying pan and fry half of the meatballs, turning occasionally, for 8–10 minutes until golden. Drain and fry the remainder. Return all the meatballs to the pan and add the cranberry glaze. Cook gently for 2–3 minutes until hot. Serve immediately.

300 g (10 oz) lean minced veal (or minced beef if preferred)
200 g (7 oz) lean minced pork
1 small onion, chopped
1 garlic clove, crushed
25 g (1 oz) breadcrumbs
1 egg yolk
3 tablespoons chopped flat leaf parsley
2 tablespoons vegetable oil
salt and pepper

Cranberry glaze
150 g (5 oz) good-quality cranberry sauce
100 ml (3½ fl oz) Chicken or Vegetable Stock (see pages 244)
2 tablespoons sweet chilli sauce
1 tablespoon lemon juice

Serves **4**
Prep time **20 minutes**
Cooking time **30 minutes**

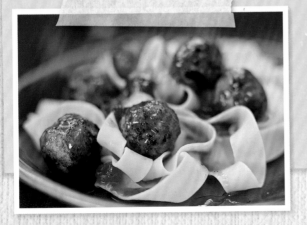

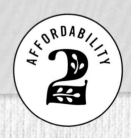

AFFORDABILITY 2

STEAK MEATLOAF

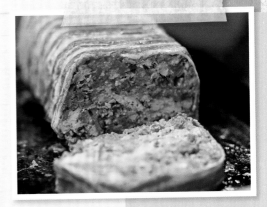

1 Scatter the red peppers and onion in a roasting tin and drizzle with the oil. Cook in a preheated oven, 200°C (400°F), Gas Mark 6, for 30 minutes until lightly roasted, then remove and chop. Reduce the oven temperature to 160°C (325°F), Gas Mark 3.

2 Use some bacon rashers to line the base and long sides of a 1 kg (2 lb) loaf tin, overlapping them slightly and letting the ends overhang the sides. Finely chop the rest of the bacon.

3 Mix together both minced meats, the chopped bacon, roasted vegetables, herbs, Worcestershire sauce, tomato paste, breadcrumbs, egg and salt and pepper.

4 Pack the mixture evenly into the tin and fold the ends of the bacon over the filling. Cover with foil, place in a roasting tin and pour in 2 cm (¾ inch) boiling water. Cook in the oven for 2 hours or until cooked through.

5 To serve hot, remove from the oven and leave the meatloaf in the tin for 15 minutes, then invert on to a serving plate. To serve cold, cool it in the tin, then remove, wrap in foil and refrigerate before serving.

2 red peppers, cored, deseeded and cut into chunks
1 red onion, sliced
3 tablespoons olive oil
300 g (10 oz) thin-cut streaky bacon rashers
500 g (1 lb) lean minced steak
250 g (8 oz) minced pork
2 tablespoons chopped oregano
2 tablespoons chopped flat leaf parsley
3 tablespoons Worcestershire sauce
2 tablespoons sun-dried tomato paste
50 g (2 oz) breadcrumbs
1 egg
salt and pepper

Serves **6**
Prep time **30 minutes, plus optional cooling**
Cooking time **2½ hours, plus standing**

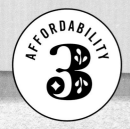

ROAST PORK LOIN
WITH CREAMY CABBAGE & LEEKS

1. Mix together the spices in a bowl, then rub over the pork. Heat 1 tablespoon of the oil in an ovenproof frying pan, add the pork and cook until browned on all sides. Transfer to a preheated oven, 180°C (350°F), Gas Mark 4, and cook for 20-25 minutes or until cooked through. Leave to rest for 2 minutes.

2. Meanwhile, cook the sweet potatoes in a saucepan of boiling water for 12-15 minutes until tender, adding the cabbage and leeks 3-4 minutes before the end of the cooking time. Drain well.

3. Heat the remaining oil in a frying pan, add the drained vegetables and fry for 7-8 minutes, stirring occasionally, until starting to turn golden. Stir in the soured cream and mustard.

4. Slice the pork and serve on top of the vegetables.

1 teaspoon ground cumin
1 teaspoon ground coriander
500 g (1 lb) pork loin, trimmed of fat
3 tablespoons olive oil
300 g (10 oz) sweet potatoes, peeled and chopped
250 g (8 oz) Savoy cabbage, shredded
3 leeks, trimmed, cleaned and sliced
3 tablespoons low-fat soured cream
2 teaspoons wholegrain mustard

Serves **4**
Prep time **10 minutes**
Cooking time **30 minutes**

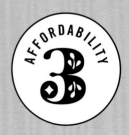

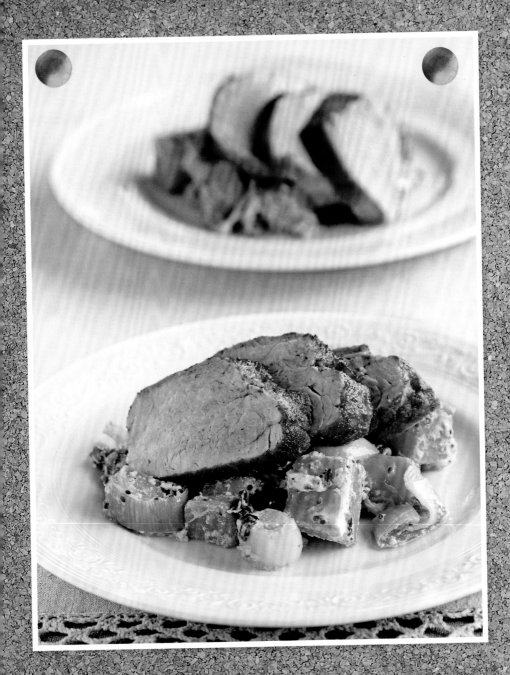

GARLICKY PORK
with Warm Butter Bean Salad

1 Mix together the oil and garlic in a bowl, then season with salt and pepper. Place the pork on a foil-lined grill rack and spoon over the garlicky oil. Cook under a preheated medium grill for about 10 minutes, turning occasionally, until golden and cooked through.

2 Meanwhile, make the salad. Heat the oil in a large frying pan, add the butter beans and tomatoes and heat through for a few minutes. Add the stock, lemon juice and parsley and season with salt and pepper. Serve with the grilled chops or steaks.

4 tablespoons olive oil
2 garlic cloves, crushed
4 lean pork chops or steaks, about 150 g (5 oz) each
salt and pepper

Salad
2 tablespoons olive oil
2 x 400 g (13 oz) cans butter beans, rinsed and drained
12 cherry tomatoes, halved
150 ml (¼ pint) Chicken Stock (see page 244)
juice of 2 lemons
2 handfuls of parsley, chopped

Serves **4**
Prep time **10 minutes**
Cooking time **10 minutes**

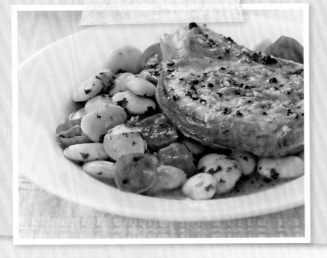

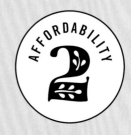

AFFORDABILITY
2

ONE-PAN SPICED PORK

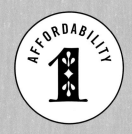

AFFORDABILITY **1**

THIS IS A GREAT DISH FOR NO-FUSS ENTERTAINING, WHEN YOU WANT TO IMPRESS YOUR HOUSEMATES. SIMPLY PLACE THE PORK CHOPS IN A ROASTING TIN WITH THE OTHER INGREDIENTS AND LEAVE THEM TO BAKE, SAFE IN THE KNOWLEDGE THAT DINNER WILL LOOK AFTER ITSELF.

1 Snip through the fat on the rind of the pork chops so that they do not curl up during cooking. Place them in a large roasting tin with the parsnips, squash and apples.

2 Crush the fennel and coriander seeds using a pestle and mortar, then mix with the garlic, turmeric, oil and honey. Season with salt and pepper, then brush the mixture over the pork and vegetables.

3 Cook in a preheated oven, 190°C (375°F), Gas Mark 5, for 35–40 minutes, turning the vegetables once, until golden brown and tender. Spoon on to plates and serve.

4 loin pork chops, about 175 g (6 oz) each
3 parsnips, cut into chunks
1 butternut squash, peeled, deseeded and thickly sliced
2 red-skinned dessert apples, cored and quartered
1 teaspoon fennel seeds
2 teaspoon coriander seeds
2 garlic cloves, chopped
1 teaspoon ground turmeric
3 tablespoons olive oil
1 tablespoon clear honey
salt and pepper

Serves **4**
Prep time **15 minutes**
Cooking time **40 minutes**

HEALTHY TIP

KEEP TABS ON YOUR ALCOHOL UNITS A cheeky pint after lectures, a few midweek drinks in the local – it all adds up. There are plenty of apps around that will tally up your drinks and help you keep on top of your recommended alcohol intake.

SPICY SAUSAGE BAKE

MAKE THIS QUICK AND EASY SUPPER DISH WITH THE MOST GARLICKY, SPICY SAUSAGES YOU CAN FIND. THEIR FLAVOUR WILL MINGLE WITH ALL THE OTHER INGREDIENTS AS THEY COOK.

1 Slice each sausage into quarters. Heat the oil in a large, heavy-based frying pan and gently fry the sausages and onion for about 10 minutes until golden, gently shaking the pan frequently.

2 Add the tomatoes, oregano and red kidney beans. Reduce the heat to its lowest setting, cover and cook gently for 10 minutes.

3 Meanwhile, cook the pasta in a large saucepan of lightly salted boiling water for about 10 minutes or until just tender. Drain and tip into the frying pan. Add half of the cheese and toss the ingredients together until mixed.

4 Tip into a 1.5 litre (2½ pint) shallow, ovenproof dish and scatter with the remaining cheese. Bake in a preheated oven, 200°C (400°F), Gas Mark 6, for 20-25 minutes or until the cheese is melting and golden.

450 g (14½ oz) Italian sausages
2 tablespoons olive oil
1 large red onion, sliced
2 x 400 g (13 oz) cans chopped tomatoes
2 tablespoons chopped oregano
400 g (13 oz) can red kidney beans, rinsed and drained
200 g (7 oz) dried fusilli pasta
175 g (6 oz) fontina cheese, grated
salt

Serves **4**
Prep time **15 minutes**
Cooking time **45 minutes**

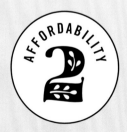

AFFORDABILITY 2

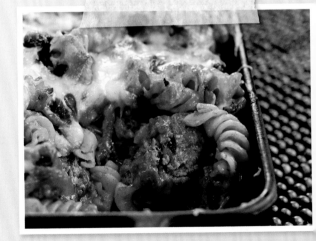

CHEESY PORK WITH PARSNIP PURÉE

1 Season the pork steaks with plenty of pepper. Heat the oil in a nonstick frying pan, add the pork steaks and fry for 2 minutes on each side until browned, then transfer to an ovenproof dish.

2 Mix together the cheese, sage, breadcrumbs and egg yolk. Divide the mixture into 4 and use to top each of the pork steaks, pressing down gently. Cook in a preheated oven, 200°C (400°F), Gas Mark 6, for 12-15 minutes until the topping is golden.

3 Meanwhile, make the parsnip purée. Place the parsnips and garlic in a saucepan of boiling water and cook for 10-12 minutes until tender. Drain, then mash with the crème fraîche and plenty of pepper. Serve with the pork steaks and steamed green beans or cabbage.

VARIATION

For chicken with breaded tomato topping, replace the pork with 4 boneless, skinless chicken breasts. Brown and lay in an ovenproof dish, as above. Make the topping as above, replacing the sage with 4 chopped sun-dried tomatoes and ¼ teaspoon dried oregano. Bake as above and serve with the parsnip purée.

4 lean pork steaks, about 125 g (4 oz) each
1 teaspoon olive oil
50 g (2 oz) crumbly cheese, such as Wensleydale or Cheshire, crumbled
1½ teaspoons chopped sage
75 g (3 oz) fresh granary breadcrumbs
1 egg yolk, beaten
pepper

Parsnip purée

625 g (1¼ lb) parsnips, chopped
2 garlic cloves, peeled
3 tablespoons half-fat crème fraîche
steamed green beans or cabbage, to serve

Serves **4**
Prep time **10 minutes**
Cooking time **20 minutes**

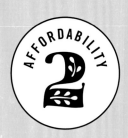

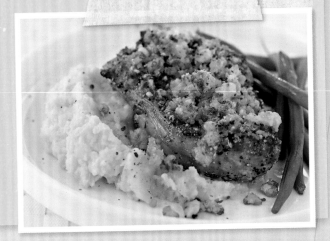

Chorizo
& HAM EGGS

1 Heat the oil in a frying pan, add the red pepper and chorizo and cook over a high heat for 2 minutes until golden. Add the tomatoes and cook for a further 2 minutes, then add the ham and spinach and cook, stirring occasionally, for 2 minutes.

2 Divide the mixture between 2 small, individual pans, if you have them (if not, continue to cook in one pan). Make wells in the tomato mixture and break an egg into each well. Cover and cook for 2-3 minutes over a medium heat until set. Serve with warm crusty bread to mop up the juices.

1 tablespoon olive oil
1 small red pepper, cored, deseeded and sliced
125 g (4 oz) chorizo sausage, thinly sliced
2 tomatoes, roughly chopped
50 g (2 oz) wafer-thin ham slices
2 handfuls of baby spinach leaves
2 large eggs
warm crusty bread, to serve

Serves **2**
Prep time **5 minutes**
Cooking time **10 minutes**

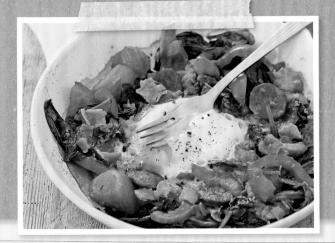

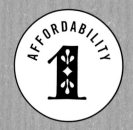

AFFORDABILITY
1

BUTTER BEAN & CHORIZO STEW

1 Heat the oil in a flameproof casserole, add the onion and garlic and fry for 1–2 minutes. Stir in the chorizo and fry until beginning to brown. Add the peppers and fry for 3 minutes.

2 Pour in the wine and allow it to bubble, then stir in the butter beans, tomatoes and tomato purée and season well with salt and pepper. Cover and simmer for 15 minutes, stirring occasionally.

3 Ladle into shallow bowls, sprinkle with the parsley to garnish and serve with crusty bread, if liked.

VARIATION
For garlic prawns with butter beans, cook the onion and garlic as above, then stir in 300 g (10 oz) raw peeled and deveined tiger prawns instead of the chorizo and fry until they just turn pink. Add the butter beans, 3 tablespoons half-fat crème fraîche and 2 handfuls of rocket and season well with salt and pepper. Heat through and serve.

1 tablespoon olive oil
1 large onion, chopped
2 garlic cloves, crushed
200 g (7 oz) chorizo sausage, sliced
1 green pepper, cored, deseeded and chopped
1 red pepper, cored, deseeded and chopped
1 small glass of red wine
2 x 400 g (13 oz) cans butter beans, rinsed and drained
400 g (13 oz) can cherry tomatoes
1 tablespoon tomato purée
salt and pepper
chopped parsley, to garnish
crusty bread, to serve (optional)

Serves **4**
Prep time **10 minutes**
Cooking time **20 minutes**

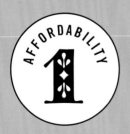

AFFORDABILITY

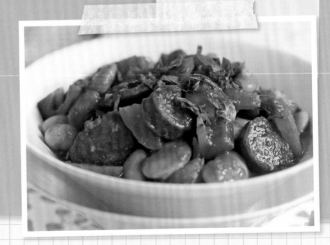

WEST INDIAN
Beef & Bean Stew

1 Heat the oil in a large, heavy-based saucepan, add the minced beef and fry, stirring, over a medium-high heat for 5–6 minutes or until browned. Add the cloves, onion and curry powder and cook for 2–3 minutes until the onion is beginning to soften, then stir in the carrots, celery, thyme, garlic and tomato purée.

2 Pour in the stock and stir well, then add the potato and beans and bring to the boil. Reduce the heat slightly and simmer for 20 minutes, uncovered, stirring occasionally, until the potatoes and beef are tender. Season to taste with salt and pepper. Ladle into bowls and serve with lemon wedges.

3 tablespoons sunflower oil
800 g (1 lb 12 oz) lean minced beef
6 whole cloves
1 onion, finely chopped
2 tablespoons medium curry powder
2 carrots, cut into 1 cm (½ inch) cubes
2 celery sticks, diced
1 tablespoon thyme leaves
2 garlic cloves, crushed
4 tablespoons tomato purée
600 ml (1 pint) beef stock
1 large potato, peeled and cut into 1 cm (½ inch) cubes
200 g (7 oz) can black beans, rinsed and drained
200 g (7 oz) can black-eyed beans, rinsed and drained
salt and pepper
lemon wedges, to serve

Serves **4–6**
Prep time **10 minutes**
Cooking time **30 minutes**

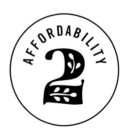
AFFORDABILITY
2

BEEF, PUMPKIN & PRUNE STEW

1 Heat the oil in a large saucepan or flameproof casserole, add the garlic, onion, pumpkin and steak and cook over a high heat for 5–10 minutes, stirring occasionally, until the beef is browned and the pumpkin is golden. Add the spices and cook for a further 1 minute.

2 Add the prunes, tomatoes and stock and bring to the boil, then reduce the heat, cover and simmer for 15 minutes, stirring occasionally, until the stew is thickened and the meat and vegetables are cooked through.

3 Scatter over the chopped coriander and stir through. Serve with steamed couscous, if liked, topped with spoonfuls of yogurt.

2 tablespoons olive oil
1 garlic clove, chopped
1 large onion, chopped
500 g (1 lb) peeled, deseeded and diced pumpkin
600 g (1 lb 5 oz) steak, such as sirloin, rump or frying, diced
2 teaspoons ground coriander
2 teaspoons ground cumin
150 g (5 oz) ready-to-eat pitted dried prunes
2 x 400 g (13 oz) cans chopped tomatoes
450 ml (¾ pint) beef stock
100 g (3½ oz) fresh coriander leaves, chopped

To serve
steamed couscous (optional)
natural yogurt

Serves **4**
Prep time **15 minutes**
Cooking time **25–30 minutes**

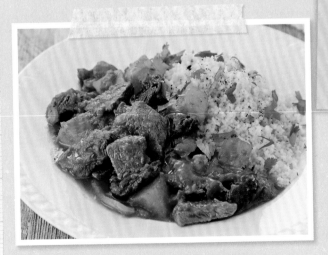

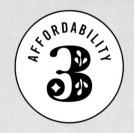

AFFORDABILITY

BAKED COD
WITH TOMATOES & OLIVES

1 Combine the tomatoes, olives, capers and thyme sprigs in a roasting tin. Nestle the cod fillets in the tin, drizzle over the oil and balsamic vinegar and season to taste with salt and pepper. Bake in a preheated oven, 200°C (400°F), Gas Mark 6, for 15 minutes until the fish is cooked through.

2 Transfer the fish, tomatoes and olives to plates. Spoon the pan juices over the fish. Garnish with thyme sprigs and serve immediately with a mixed green leaf salad, if liked.

VARIATION
For steamed cod with lemon, arrange a cod fillet on each of 4 x 30 cm (12 inch) squares of foil. Top each with ½ teaspoon finely grated lemon rind, a squeeze of lemon juice, 1 tablespoon extra virgin olive oil and salt and pepper to taste. Fold the edges of the foil together to form parcels, transfer to a baking sheet and cook in a preheated oven, 200°C (400°F), Gas Mark 6, for 15 minutes. Remove and leave to rest for 5 minutes. Open the parcels and serve sprinkled with chopped parsley.

250 g (8 oz) cherry tomatoes, halved
100 g (3½ oz) pitted black olives
2 tablespoons capers, drained
4 thyme sprigs, plus extra to garnish
4 cod fillets, about 175 g (6 oz) each
2 tablespoons extra virgin olive oil
2 tablespoons balsamic vinegar
salt and pepper
mixed green leaf salad, to serve (optional)

Serves **4**
Prep time **5 minutes**
Cooking time **15 minutes**

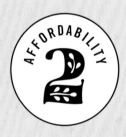

AFFORDABILITY 2

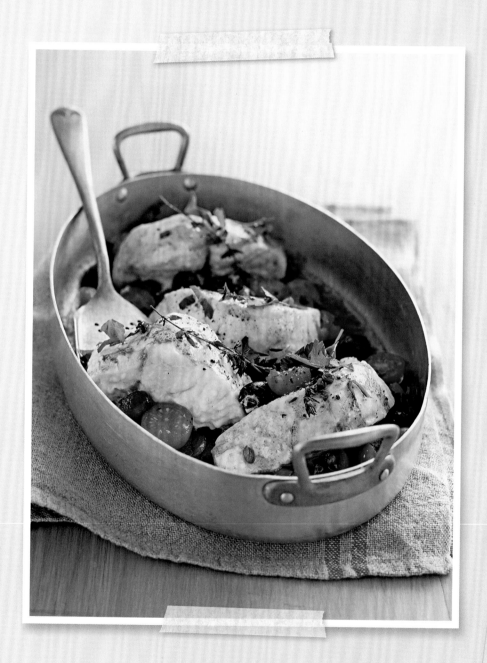

HADDOCK
WITH POACHED EGGS

1 Place the potatoes in a saucepan of boiling water and cook for 12-15 minutes until tender. Drain, lightly crush with a fork, then stir through the spring onions, crème fraîche and watercress and season well with pepper. Keep warm.

2 Put the fish and milk in a large frying pan with the bay leaf. Bring to the boil, then cover and simmer for 5-6 minutes until the fish is cooked through. Remove from the heat and let stand while you poach the eggs.

3 Bring a saucepan of water to the boil, swirl the water with a spoon and crack in an egg, allowing the white to wrap around the yolk. Simmer for 3 minutes, then remove and keep warm. Repeat with the remaining eggs.

4 Serve the drained poached haddock on top of the crushed potatoes, topped with the poached eggs.

VARIATION

For a warm haddock, asparagus and egg salad, replace the new potatoes with 325 g (11 oz) asparagus and cook in boiling water for 5 minutes, then drain. Place in a bowl with the spring onions, crème fraîche and watercress, adding the leaves of a Little Gem lettuce and 1 tablespoon extra virgin olive oil; toss to mix. Poach the haddock as above, remove from the milk with a slotted spoon and break into flakes. Toss the fish in the asparagus salad and divide between 4 plates. Serve with a poached egg on top, prepared as above.

750 g (1½ lb) new potatoes
4 spring onions, sliced
2 tablespoons half-fat crème fraîche
75 g (3 oz) watercress
4 smoked haddock fillets, about 150 g (5 oz) each
150 ml (¼ pint) milk
1 bay leaf
4 eggs
pepper

Serves **4**
Prep time **10 minutes**
Cooking time **30 minutes**

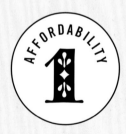

AFFORDABILITY
1

SMOKED MACKEREL KEDGEREE

1. Place the eggs in a small saucepan of boiling water and cook them for 7 minutes. Drain, run under cold water, then shell them and cut into quarters.

2. Meanwhile, melt the butter in a frying pan, add the smoked mackerel, rice and curry powder and toss together until everything is warmed through and the rice is evenly coated.

3. Stir in the lemon juice, parsley and the quartered boiled eggs and serve immediately.

3 large eggs
25 g (1 oz) butter
375 g (12 oz) smoked mackerel, skinned and flaked
375 g (12 oz) cooked basmati rice
1 teaspoon mild curry powder
4 tablespoons lemon juice
4 tablespoons chopped parsley

Serves **4**
Prep time **5 minutes**
Cooking time **15 minutes**

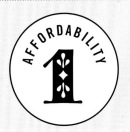
AFFORDABILITY 1

STUDENT TIP

BAG A BARGAIN If you have space in your freezer, make the most of supermarket bargains and tuck them away for when the budget is straining.

SWEET GLAZED MACKEREL
WITH CRISPY KALE & NOODLES

1 Put the kale in a roasting tin and drizzle with 1 teaspoon of the oil. Bake in a preheated oven, 200°C (400°F), Gas Mark 6, for 6-8 minutes until crisped.

2 Pat the mackerel dry on kitchen paper and cut in half. Bring a saucepan of water to the boil and cook the noodles for 2-3 minutes until softened.

3 Meanwhile, heat the remaining oil in a small frying pan and fry the mackerel, skin side up, for 2 minutes. Turn the pieces and cook for a further couple of minutes until cooked through.

4 Drain the noodles and return to the pan. Stir in the kale and transfer to a serving plate. Arrange the fish on top.

5 Add the garlic to the frying pan and cook for 30 seconds. Add the lime juice, chilli sauce, sugar and water to the saucepan and heat through. Pour over the fish and serve.

50 g (2 oz) kale
2 teaspoons oil
1 large mackerel fillet (skin on), defrosted if frozen, about 125 g (4 oz)
50 g (2 oz) wholewheat noodles
1 small garlic clove, thinly sliced
1 tablespoon lime juice
2 tablespoons sweet chilli sauce
1 teaspoon light muscovado or caster sugar
2 tablespoons water

Serves **1**
Prep time **5 minutes**
Cooking time **10 minutes**

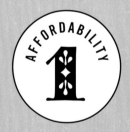

ONE-POT FISH ROAST WITH AÏOLI

1. Put the beetroot, potatoes and onion in a small roasting tin with the garlic clove. Drizzle with the oil and season with a little salt and pepper, then roast in a preheated oven 220°C (425°F), Gas Mark 7, for about 30 minutes, turning once during cooking. Add the courgette slices to the tin and return to the oven for a further 20 minutes or until the vegetables are tender and lightly roasted. Remove the garlic clove once it's soft and tender.

2. Mix the rosemary or thyme with the lemon rind and plenty of pepper. Score the skin side of the trout with a sharp knife. Rub the herb mixture over both sides of the fish and add to the tin, skin side up. Roast for a further 10-15 minutes until the fish is cooked through.

3. Scoop out the soft pulp of the roasted garlic clove and mix it with the mayonnaise.

4. Transfer the fish and vegetables to a serving plate, spooning over any pan juices. Serve with the aïoli.

1 raw beetroot, about 150 g (5 oz), scrubbed and cut into wedges
100 g (3½ oz) new potatoes
1 red onion, cut into wedges
1 whole garlic clove, unpeeled
2 teaspoons olive oil
1 courgette, sliced
½ teaspoon finely chopped rosemary or thyme
finely grated rind of ½ lemon
1 trout fillet (skin on), about 175-200 g (6-7 oz)
2 tablespoons mayonnaise
salt and pepper

Serves **1**
Prep time **10 minutes**
Cooking time **1 hour**

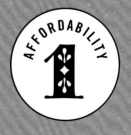

AFFORDABILITY 1

Quick Tuna FISHCAKES

MOST OF US HAVE A COUPLE OF CANS OF TUNA IN THE STORECUPBOARD, BUT SOMETIMES THE IDEAS ABOUT WHAT TO DO WITH THEM GET A BIT TIRED. HERE'S A QUICK AND DELICIOUS RECIPE TO TRY OUT – SEE IF YOU AND YOUR HOUSEMATES LIKE IT.

1 Cook the potatoes in a saucepan of lightly salted boiling water for 10 minutes or until tender. Drain well, mash and cool slightly.

2 Flake the tuna. Beat the tuna, cheese, spring onions, garlic, thyme and egg into the mashed potatoes. Season to taste with cayenne, salt and pepper.

3 Divide the mixture into 4 even portions and shape each one into a thick patty. Season the flour with salt and pepper, then dust the patties all over with the flour.

4 Heat a shallow layer of vegetable oil in a frying pan until hot, then fry the fishcakes for 5 minutes on each side or until crisp and golden. Serve hot with a mixed green salad and mayonnaise.

250 g (8 oz) baking potatoes, peeled and diced
2 x 200 g (7 oz) cans tuna in olive oil, drained
50 g (2 oz) Cheddar cheese, grated
4 spring onions, finely chopped
1 small garlic clove, crushed
2 teaspoons dried thyme
1 small egg, beaten
½ teaspoon cayenne pepper
4 tablespoons plain flour
vegetable oil, for frying
salt and pepper

To serve
mixed green salad
mayonnaise

Serves **4**
Prep time **15 minutes**
Cooking time **20 minutes**

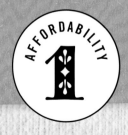

AFFORDABILITY
1

RED SALMON
& ROASTED VEGETABLES

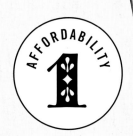

1 Mix together the aubergine, red peppers, onions and garlic in a bowl with the oil and oregano and season well with salt and pepper. Spread the vegetables out in a single layer in a nonstick roasting tin and roast in a preheated oven, 220°C (425°F), Gas Mark 7, for 25 minutes or until the vegetables are just cooked.

2 Transfer the vegetables to a warmed serving dish and gently toss in the salmon and olives. Serve warm or at room temperature, garnished with basil leaves.

ACCOMPANIMENT TIP
For rocket and cucumber couscous to serve with the salmon and vegetables, put 200 g (7 oz) instant couscous in a large, heatproof bowl. Season well with salt and pepper and pour over boiling hot water to just cover the couscous. Cover and leave to stand for 10-12 minutes until all the water has been absorbed. Meanwhile, finely chop 4 spring onions, halve, deseed and chop ½ cucumber and chop 75 g (3 oz) rocket. Fluff up the couscous grains with a fork and tip into a serving dish. Stir in the prepared ingredients along with 2 tablespoons olive oil and 1 tablespoon lemon juice. Toss well to mix, then serve with the salmon and vegetables.

1 aubergine, cut into bite-sized pieces
2 red peppers, cored, deseeded and cut into bite-sized pieces
2 red onions, quartered
1 garlic clove, crushed
4 tablespoons olive oil
pinch of dried oregano
200 g (7 oz) can red salmon, drained and flaked
100 g (3½ oz) pitted black olives
salt and pepper
basil leaves, to garnish

Serves **4**
Prep time **10 minutes**
Cooking time **25 minutes**

Good Grains, Beans & Pulses

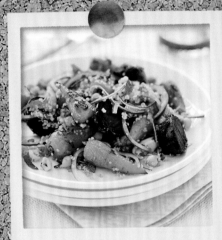

ROASTED ROOTS & QUINOA SALAD

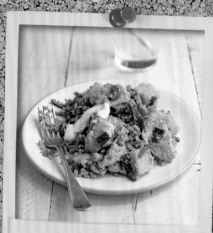

CURRIED CHICKEN
& COUSCOUS SALAD

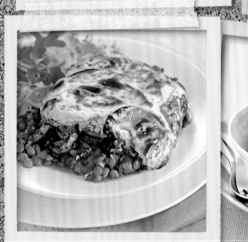

LENTIL MOUSSAKA

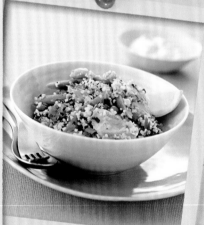

SALMON &
BULGAR WHEAT PILAF

CHICKEN
WITH HERBY QUINOA & LEMON

1   Cook the quinoa in a saucepan of lightly salted boiling water for 15 minutes until tender, then drain.

2   Meanwhile, heat the oil in a large frying pan, add the onion and cook, stirring, for 5 minutes to soften. Add the garlic, chicken, coriander and cumin and cook for a further 8-10 minutes, stirring occasionally, until the chicken is cooked.

3   Season the quinoa with salt and pepper. Add the chicken mixture, cranberries, apricots, herbs and lemon rind. Stir well and serve warm or cold.

VARIATION

For chicken and apricot Moroccan couscous, put 100 g (3½ oz) Moroccan-flavoured couscous in a bowl, cover with boiling water, cover the bowl with clingfilm and leave to stand for 8 minutes. When all the water has been absorbed, stir in 250 g (8 oz) chopped cooked chicken, 125 g (4 oz) ready-to-eat dried apricots and a 220 g (7½ oz) can chickpeas, rinsed and drained.

200 g (7 oz) quinoa, rinsed and drained
1 tablespoon olive oil
1 onion, chopped
1 garlic clove, crushed
4 boneless, skinless chicken breasts, sliced
1 teaspoon ground coriander
½ teaspoon ground cumin
50 g (2 oz) dried cranberries
75 g (3 oz) ready-to-eat dried apricots, chopped
4 tablespoons chopped parsley
4 tablespoons chopped mint
finely grated rind of 1 lemon
salt and pepper

Serves **4**
Prep time **15 minutes**
Cooking time **15 minutes**

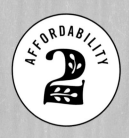

AFFORDABILITY 2

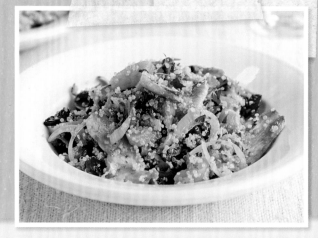

CHARGRILLED CHICKEN
WITH SALSA & FRUITY COUSCOUS

1 Place the chicken in a non-metallic container, pour over the vinegar and turn to coat. Cover and leave to marinate for 5 minutes.

2 Place the couscous in a heatproof bowl, pour over the slightly cooled boiled water and season with a little salt. Cover and leave to absorb the water for 10 minutes.

3 Meanwhile, heat 1 tablespoon of the oil in a large frying pan or griddle pan and cook the chicken over a medium heat, turning once, for 10-12 minutes until browned and cooked through.

4 While the chicken is cooking, make the salsa by mixing together the avocado, tomato, 1 tablespoon of the remaining olive oil and 1 tablespoon of the coriander in a bowl.

5 Stir the remaining tablespoon of olive oil into the couscous, then add the raisins, pumpkin seeds and remaining coriander and toss again. Serve on plates topped with the chicken, with the salsa spooned over.

4 boneless, skinless chicken
    breasts, about 150 g (5 oz) each
6 tablespoons balsamic vinegar
175 g (6 oz) couscous
350 ml (12 fl oz) boiled water,
    slightly cooled
3 tablespoons olive oil
1 ripe avocado, peeled, stoned
    and roughly chopped
1 large tomato, roughly chopped
5 tablespoons chopped fresh
    coriander
50 g (2 oz) raisins
4 tablespoons pumpkin seeds
salt

Serves **4**
Prep time **15 minutes, plus marinating**
Cooking time **15 minutes**

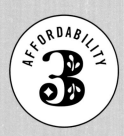

AFFORDABILITY
3

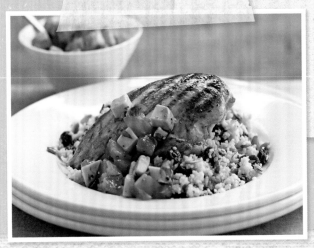

Spiced Chicken
WITH MIXED GRAINS

1 Heat the oil in a saucepan and add the chicken and onion. Cook, stirring frequently for 5 minutes. Add the garlic, turmeric, chilli flakes and stock and bring to a gentle simmer. Cover and cook gently for 10 minutes.

2 Stir in the swede, wheat grains, quinoa and mustard and cook gently for a further 30 minutes, stirring occasionally, until the grains are tender and the juices are thickened. Season to taste with salt and pepper.

3 Spoon into serving bowls and serve topped with spoonfuls of Greek yogurt.

1 tablespoon vegetable oil
450 g (14½ oz) boneless, skinless chicken thighs, cut into chunks
1 onion, chopped
2 garlic cloves, crushed
¼ teaspoon ground turmeric
¼ teaspoon dried chilli flakes
500 ml (17 fl oz) Chicken or Vegetable Stock (see page 244)
½ small swede, about 300 g (10 oz), peeled and cut into small chunks
50 g (2 oz) wheat grains
25 g (1 oz) quinoa, rinsed and drained
1 teaspoon wholegrain mustard
salt and pepper
0%-fat Greek yogurt, to serve

Serves **2**
Prep time **10 minutes**
Cooking time **45 minutes**

STUDENT TIP

DON'T FALL FOR CONVENIENCE If you're organized and have a weekly meal plan you should be able to buy the majority of your groceries in one big, online weekly shop. If you end up wandering down to the corner shop in your onesie every evening to stock up on staples, you'll soon feel the pinch in your pocket.

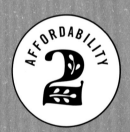

AFFORDABILITY 2

WINTER SPICED COUSCOUS

 Vegan

1 Mix together the carrot, onion and olive oil in a large, microwave-proof mug. Microwave on full power for 3 minutes, stirring after 2 minutes.

2 Stir in the spices, couscous, bouillon powder, coriander and chickpeas, then stir in the boiling water. Microwave on full power for a further 1 minute. Stir to combine and then serve.

1 small carrot, cut into small dice
1 small red onion, chopped
2 teaspoons olive oil
good pinch each of ground allspice and ground cloves
50 g (2 oz) couscous
½ teaspoon vegetable bouillon powder
1 tablespoon chopped fresh coriander
50 g (2 oz) canned chickpeas, rinsed and drained
50 ml (2 fl oz) boiling water

Serves **1**
Prep time **10 minutes**
Cooking time **4 minutes**

STUDENT TIP

DON'T BE A BRAND SNOB Try swapping your staple purchases for the supermarket own-brand equivalents — you'll save a fortune and chances are you won't notice the difference when it comes to taste.

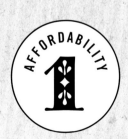

Salmon
& Bulgar Wheat Pilaf

1. Cook the salmon in a steamer or microwave on full power for about 10 minutes. Alternatively, wrap it in foil and cook in a preheated oven, 180°C (350°F), Gas Mark 4, for 15 minutes.

2. Meanwhile, cook the bulgar wheat according to the packet instructions and cook the peas and beans in a saucepan of boiling water for about 5 minutes. Alternatively, cook the peas and beans in the steamer with the salmon.

3. Flake the salmon and mix it into the bulgar wheat with the peas and beans. Fold in the chives and parsley and season to taste with salt and pepper. Serve immediately with the lemon wedges and yogurt.

VARIATION

For ham and bulgar wheat pilaf, lightly pan-fry 300 g (10 oz) diced lean cooked ham instead of the salmon. Replace the runner beans with the same quantity of shelled broad beans and fold in 2 tablespoons chopped mint along with the chives and parsley.

475 g (15 oz) boneless, skinless salmon fillets
250 g (8 oz) bulgar wheat
75 g (3 oz) frozen peas
200 g (7 oz) runner beans, chopped
2 tablespoons snipped chives
2 tablespoons chopped flat leaf parsley
salt and pepper

To serve
lemon wedges
low-fat natural yogurt

Serves **4**
Prep time **10 minutes**
Cooking time **15-20 minutes**

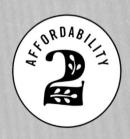

AFFORDABILITY
2

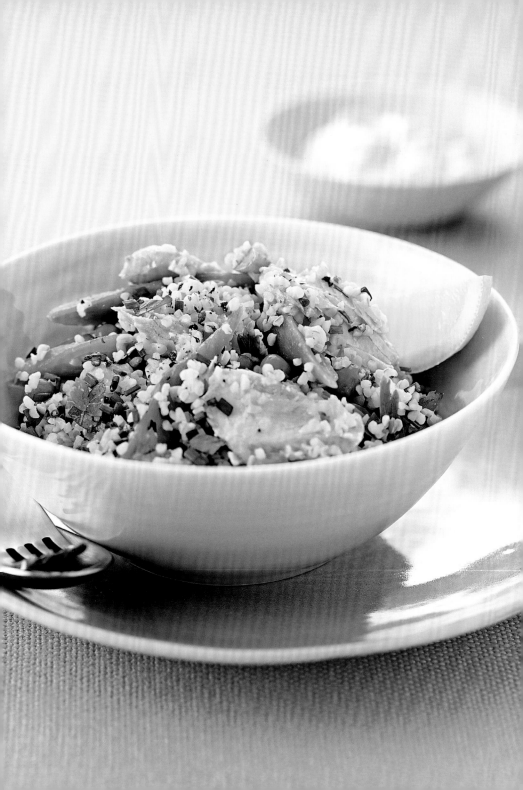

RED KIDNEY BEAN & AUBERGINE PILAF

Vegan

1 Pour the water into a large saucepan and bring to the boil. Add the rice and turmeric and stir well to prevent the rice from sticking. Cover and simmer for 30 minutes without stirring. Remove from the heat.

2 Meanwhile, heat the oil in a nonstick frying pan, add the onion, garlic, celery, green pepper and aubergine and cook gently for 3 minutes without browning. Add the tomatoes and mushrooms, stir well and cook for 3–4 minutes.

3 Stir the beans and the vegetable mixture into the rice, cover and cook very gently for 10 minutes.

4 Remove from the heat and leave to rest for 5 minutes. Stir in the parsley and season to taste with pepper.

VARIATION
Add 550 g (1 lb 4 oz) cooked and chopped boneless, skinless chicken breasts before the tomatoes and mushrooms, for an alternative non-vegan supper.

450 ml (¾ pint) water
250 g (8 oz) long-grain brown rice
½ teaspoon ground turmeric
1 tablespoon vegetable oil
1 large onion, finely chopped
1 garlic clove, finely chopped
1 celery stick, finely chopped
1 green pepper, cored, deseeded and chopped
1 aubergine, diced
2 tomatoes, skinned and chopped
125 g (4 oz) mushrooms, trimmed and sliced
1 x 200 g (7 oz) can red kidney beans, rinsed and drained
2 tablespoons chopped parsley
pepper

Serves **4**
Prep time **15 minutes**
Cooking time **40 minutes, plus resting**

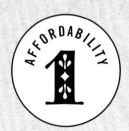

HEALTHY TIP

Beans are a good source of protein, especially when they are served with a cereal food such as rice, bread or pasta. They are low in fat, high in fibre and rich in many nutrients, providing iron, zinc, calcium, folate and soluble fibre.

PASTA WITH SPICY LENTILS

THIS DISH HAS A SLIGHTLY SWEET AND SOUR FLAVOUR, WHICH GIVES AN APPETIZING LIFT TO THE EARTHY FLAVOUR OF THE LENTILS. USE ANY DRIED PASTA SHAPES WITH THIS DISH.

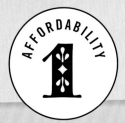

1 Put the lentils in a saucepan with the stock, bay leaves and onion. Bring to the boil, reduce the heat to its lowest setting, cover and cook gently for about 20-25 minutes or until the lentils are tender and the stock has been absorbed or almost absorbed.

2 Meanwhile, bring a separate large saucepan of lightly salted water to the boil. Add the pasta, return to the boil and cook for about 8-10 minutes or until just tender.

3 While the pasta is cooking, heat 1 tablespoon of the oil in a frying pan and fry the courgettes until golden. Add the tomatoes and fry for a further 1 minute to soften slightly.

4 Beat the remaining oil with the chilli, honey, mustard and lemon juice in a small bowl.

5 Drain the pasta and return to the pan. Drain the lentils of any unabsorbed stock and tip them into the pasta pan, discarding the bay leaves and onion quarters. Add the courgettes, tomatoes, dressing and herbs and toss all the ingredients together. Check and adjust the seasoning to taste and serve warm.

200 g (7 oz) black or Puy lentils, rinsed
1 litre (1¾ pints) Vegetable Stock (see page 244)
3 bay leaves
1 onion, quartered
250 g (8 oz) plain or spinach-flavoured dried pasta
5 tablespoons mild olive oil
2 small courgettes, thinly sliced
250 g (8 oz) cherry tomatoes, halved
1 red chilli, thinly sliced
2 tablespoons clear honey
2 tablespoons wholegrain mustard
1 tablespoon lemon juice
25 g (1 oz) mixed herbs, such as parsley, mint and chives, finely chopped
salt and pepper

Serves **4**
Prep time **15 minutes**
Cooking time **20-25 minutes**

TAGLIATELLE
WITH SPICY PEA FRITTERS

1 Put the split peas in a large bowl, cover with cold water and leave to soak overnight. Drain and put in a saucepan. Cover with fresh cold water, bring to the boil, and cook for about 25 minutes until tender. Drain.

2 Tip the cooked split peas into a blender or food processor with the onion, breadcrumbs, garlic, cumin, chilli flakes, mint sprigs, egg and salt and pepper and process to a smooth paste. Divide and shape the paste firmly into small balls, each about 2.5 cm (1 inch) in diameter.

3 Bring a large saucepan of lightly salted water to the boil, add the pasta, return to the boil and cook for about 10 minutes until just tender.

4 Meanwhile, heat half of the oil with the butter in a large frying pan. Add the pea fritters and fry gently, stirring, for 5 minutes or until golden. You may need to do this in batches.

5 Drain the pasta and return it to the saucepan. Stir in the peppers, coriander, pea fritters and remaining oil and mix together gently before serving.

300 g (10 oz) yellow split peas
1 onion, roughly chopped
25 g (1 oz) white or wholemeal breadcrumbs
2 garlic cloves, chopped
1 tablespoon crushed cumin seeds
¾ teaspoon dried chilli flakes
several sprigs of mint
1 egg
200 g (7 oz) dried tagliatelle
8 tablespoons lemon-infused olive oil
25 g (1 oz) butter
200 g (7 oz) roasted red peppers in oil (from a jar), drained and thinly sliced
4 tablespoons chopped fresh coriander
salt and pepper

Serves **4**
Prep time **30 minutes, plus overnight soaking**
Cooking time **40 minutes**

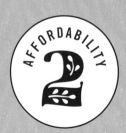

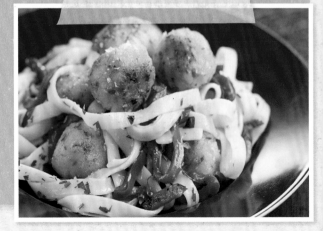

SPINACH DHAL

NO INDIAN MEAL IS COMPLETE WITHOUT A BOWL OF SPICY LENTIL DHAL, WHICH IS ONE OF THE STAPLE DISHES EATEN THROUGHOUT THE COUNTRY. THIS ONE USES FRESH, TENDER BABY SPINACH FOR EXTRA FLAVOUR, COLOUR AND TEXTURE.

1 Place the lentils in a large saucepan with the water, turmeric and ginger. Bring to the boil. Skim off any scum that forms on the surface. Lower the heat and cook gently for 20 minutes, stirring occasionally. Stir in the spinach and chopped coriander and cook for 8-10 minutes.

2 Heat the oil in a small, nonstick frying pan until hot, then add the garlic, cumin and mustard seeds, ground cumin, ground coriander and red chilli. Stir-fry over a high heat for 2-3 minutes, then tip this mixture into the lentils. Stir to mix well, season lightly with salt, then serve immediately with boiled rice or warm naan bread.

250 g (8 oz) red lentils, rinsed and drained
1.2 litres (2 pints) water
1 teaspoon ground turmeric
1 teaspoon peeled and finely grated fresh root ginger
100 g (3½ oz) baby spinach leaves, chopped
large handful of fresh coriander leaves, chopped
2 teaspoons light olive oil
5 garlic cloves, thinly sliced
2 teaspoons cumin seeds
2 teaspoons mustard seeds
1 tablespoon ground cumin
1 teaspoon ground coriander
1 red chilli, finely chopped
salt
Boiled Rice (see page 246) or warm naan bread, to serve

Serves **4**
Prep time **10 minutes**
Cooking time **35 minutes**

HEALTHY TIP

Both lentils and spinach are an excellent source of iron, making this dish a real iron-booster. Lentils are also a great source of fibre and protein, so dhal is a great choice for a vegetarian meal.

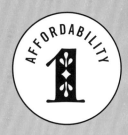

CURRIED CHICKEN COUSCOUS SALAD

1 Place the couscous in a bowl and pour over enough boiling water to just cover. Season lightly with salt, cover and set aside for 20 minutes to swell.

2 Meanwhile, heat the oil in a frying pan and cook the onion and chicken slices over a high heat for 5 minutes, turning occasionally. Reduce the heat, add the spring onions and cook for a further 3–4 minutes until softened and cooked through. Remove from the heat and keep warm.

3 In a separate frying pan, heat the curry paste over a low heat until softened, adding the water to loosen. Drain the couscous (if needed) and transfer to the pan with the curry paste. Toss and stir to coat and heat, for about 2 minutes.

4 Combine the cooked chicken and onion with the curried couscous. Add the mango and coriander, if using, and toss again before serving with spoonfuls of natural yogurt, if liked.

125 g (4 oz) barley couscous (wheat couscous would also be fine to use)
3 tablespoons olive oil
1 red onion, sliced
375 g (12 oz) boneless, skinless chicken breasts, thinly sliced
bunch of spring onions, cut into strips
4 tablespoons korma curry paste
2 tablespoons water
1 ripe mango, peeled, stoned and cut into chunks
4 tablespoons chopped fresh coriander (optional)
salt
natural yogurt, to serve (optional)

....

Serves **4**
Prep time **15 minutes, plus soaking**
Cooking time **15 minutes**

....

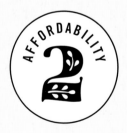

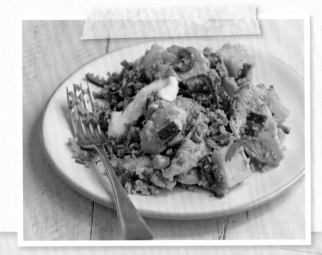

Minted Rice with Tomato & SPROUTED BEANS

Vegan

THE SPROUTED BEANS IN THIS LIGHT AND FRESH STIR-FRIED RICE DISH GIVE IT A CRUNCHY BITE, WHILE THE GENEROUS ADDITION OF GARLIC GIVES A RICH, AROMATIC FLAVOUR

1 Heat the oil in a large, nonstick wok or frying pan until hot, then add the spring onions and garlic and stir-fry for 2–3 minutes.

2 Add the cooked rice and continue to stir-fry over a high heat for 3–4 minutes. Stir in the tomatoes and mixed sprouted beans and stir-fry for a further 2–3 minutes or until warmed through.

3 Remove from the heat, season to taste with salt and pepper, then stir in the chopped mint. Serve immediately.

2 tablespoons light olive oil
6 spring onions, very thinly sliced
2 garlic cloves, finely chopped
750 g (1½ lb) cooked, cooled
   basmati rice
2 plum tomatoes, finely chopped
250 g (8 oz) mixed sprouted
   beans, such as aduki, mung,
   lentil and chickpea sprouts
small handful of mint leaves,
   chopped
salt and pepper

Serves **4**
Prep time **10 minutes**
Cooking time **8–10 minutes**

HEALTHY TIP

Sprouted beans are a living food, packed with valuable vitamins, minerals and health-giving phytochemicals. They are widely available in large supermarkets and health food stores, or you can sprout your own at home.

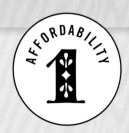

AFFORDABILITY
1

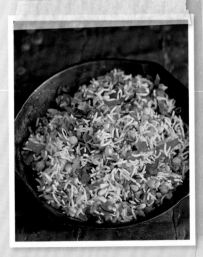

Spicy Lentils & Chickpeas

1 Heat the oil in a heavy-based saucepan over a medium heat, add the onion, garlic, celery and green pepper and fry gently, stirring occasionally, for 10-12 minutes or until softened and beginning to colour.

2 Stir in the lentils and spices and cook for 2-3 minutes, stirring frequently. Add the tomato purée, stock and chickpeas and bring to the boil. Reduce the heat, cover and simmer gently for about 20 minutes until the lentils collapse. Season to taste with salt and pepper.

3 Ladle into bowls and garnish with the chopped coriander. Serve immediately with boiled rice and spiced yogurt (see Tip below), if liked.

ACCOMPANIMENT TIP

For cooling, spiced yogurt to serve as an accompaniment, mix together 200 ml (7 fl oz) fat-free natural yogurt, 2 tablespoons lemon juice and ½ teaspoon garam masala in a small bowl. Fold in ½ small, deseeded and grated cucumber, then season to taste with salt and pepper. Serve sprinkled with 1 tablespoon chopped fresh coriander.

1 tablespoon groundnut oil
1 onion, finely chopped
2 garlic cloves, thinly sliced
2 celery sticks, diced
1 green pepper, cored, deseeded and chopped
150 g (5 oz) split red lentils, rinsed and drained
2 teaspoons garam masala
1 teaspoon cumin seeds
½ teaspoon hot chilli powder
1 teaspoon ground coriander
2 tablespoons tomato purée
750 ml (1¼ pints) Vegetable Stock (see page 244)
400 g (13 oz) can chickpeas, rinsed and drained
salt and pepper
2 tablespoons chopped fresh coriander, to garnish

To serve (optional)
Boiled rice (see page 247)
spiced yogurt (see Tip)

Serves **4**
Prep time **15 minutes**
Cooking time **35 minutes**

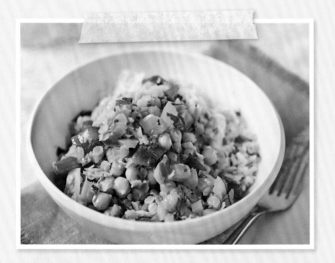

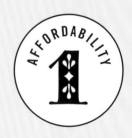

PUY LENTIL STEW
WITH GARLIC & HERB BREAD

1 Heat the oil in a large, heavy-based saucepan and cook the peppers, onion, garlic and fennel over a medium-high heat, stirring frequently, for 5 minutes until softened and lightly browned. Stir in the lentils, stock and wine and bring to the boil, then reduce the heat and simmer, stirring occasionally, for 25 minutes until the lentils are tender.

2 Meanwhile, for the garlic bread, beat the butter with the garlic and thyme in a bowl and season with a little salt and pepper. Cut the baguette into thick slices, almost all the way through but leaving the base attached. Spread the butter thickly over each slice, then wrap the baguette in foil and cook in a preheated oven, 200°C (400°F), Gas Mark 6, for 15 minutes.

3 Serve the hot stew, ladled into serving bowls, with the torn hot garlic and herb bread on the side for mopping up the juices.

4 tablespoons olive oil
1 red pepper, cored, deseeded and cut into chunks
1 green pepper, cored, deseeded and cut into chunks
1 red onion, roughly chopped
1 garlic clove, sliced
1 fennel bulb, trimmed and sliced
250 g (8 oz) Puy lentils, rinsed
600 ml (1 pint) Vegetable Stock (see page 244)
300 ml (½ pint) red wine

Garlic bread
50 g (2 oz) butter, softened
1 garlic clove, crushed
2 tablespoons roughly chopped thyme leaves
1 wholemeal French baguette
salt and pepper

Serves **4**
Prep time **15 minutes**
Cooking time **35 minutes**

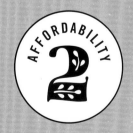

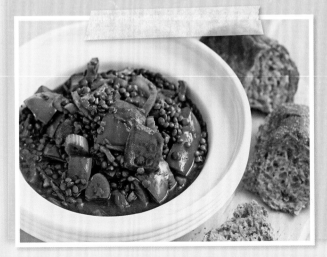

FREE WAYS TO GET FIT

You don't need to splash out on an expensive monthly gym membership to stay fit and healthy. If your budget won't stretch to paying for your stretches, there are plenty of ways you can tone up in your downtime.

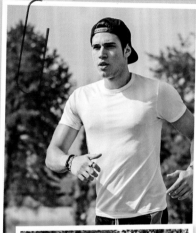

RUN WILD

If you have a pair of trackies and trainers, you can start running straight away. It's easy to fit into uni life, as you're not pinned down to certain days and times. Begin with a gentle jog around the block and slowly build up to longer runs.

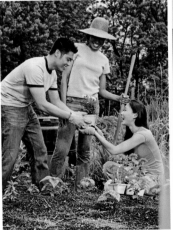

PULL ON YOUR GARDENING GLOVES

Got a garden? If you're lucky enough to have some outside space in your uni digs, chances are it won't be entered into any competitions at Chelsea Flower Show. It might be a stereotype but students don't tend to get overexcited about borders and bedding plants. You might clear a space in the undergrowth for a disposable BBQ but the garden will be largely unloved. But gardening is great exercise and there's the added advantage of having something to show for your efforts.

WORKOUT IN THE LIBRARY

Well not literally… but you can borrow exercise DVDs for a minimal fee and have a workout in the privacy of your living room. Alternatively, there are literally thousands of routines for every imaginable type of keep fit available on the internet – just don't spend more time surfing than exercising.

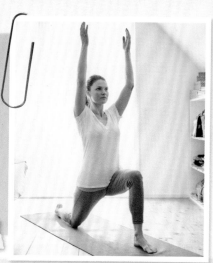

SAY BYE TO THE BUS

Walking is a great way to get fit without breaking into a sweat. A brisk 20-minute walk in the morning will set you up for the day and give you time to get your thoughts in order. So, if you usually travel into college by bus, put your fare back in your pocket and use your legs instead. It's free, you don't need any special equipment and it gets you from A to B… what's not to like?

HIT THE DANCE FLOOR

If you're used to sedentary social activities, it might be time to get your butt off the bar stool and start throwing some shapes. Dancing burns plenty of calories but hopefully you'll be having such a good time that you won't notice.

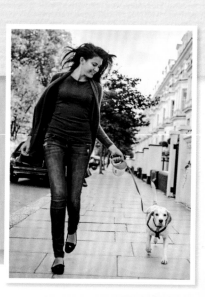

ADOPT A DOG

You're unlikely to have a dog living at your digs – landlords tend to be a bit fussy when it comes to pets. However, you could offer your services as a dog walker and benefit from plenty of exercise and fresh air, as well as earning a bit of money.

ROAST TOMATO & BROAD
BEAN TABBOULEH

 Vegan

1. Arrange the tomato halves, cut side up, in a roasting tin. Sprinkle with the oregano, sugar and a little pepper. Drizzle with 1 tablespoon of the oil and roast in a preheated oven, 180°C (350°F), Gas Mark 4, for 1 hour.

2. Meanwhile, put the bulgar wheat in a saucepan with the bouillon powder and cover with the water. Bring to a gentle simmer, cover with a lid and cook for 15 minutes until the bulgar wheat is tender and the water absorbed. Remove from the heat, drain off any excess water, then turn into a bowl. Stir in the cumin and pumpkin or sunflower seeds. Leave to cool.

3. Cook the broad beans in a small saucepan of boiling water for 3 minutes. Drain, then add to the bulgar wheat mixture with the parsley, the remaining oil and the lemon juice. Stir in the roast tomatoes along with any juices and serve.

500 g (1 lb) tomatoes, halved
good pinch of dried oregano
½ teaspoon caster sugar
2 tablespoons olive oil
100 g (3½ oz) bulgar wheat, rinsed
1 teaspoon vegetable bouillon powder
600 ml (1 pint) water
1 teaspoon cumin seeds
25 g (1 oz) pumpkin or sunflower seeds
100 g (3½ oz) frozen baby broad beans
25 g (1 oz) parsley, chopped
squeeze of lemon juice
pepper

Serves **2**
Prep time **10 minutes**
Cooking time **1 hour**

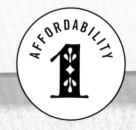

AFFORDABILITY 1

GRILLED HALOUMI
WITH WARM COUSCOUS SALAD

1   Place the couscous in a bowl and add enough boiling water to cover by 1 cm (½ inch). Season lightly with salt and leave the couscous to absorb the water for 10 minutes.

2   Meanwhile, heat 3 tablespoons of the oil in a large frying pan and cook the onions and two-thirds of the chilli over a medium heat, stirring, for 4-5 minutes until softened. Add the chickpeas and tomatoes and cook over a high heat, stirring occasionally, for 3 minutes until the chickpeas are heated through and the tomatoes are softened but still retaining their shape.

3   Meanwhile, mix the remaining oil and chilli with the herbs in a shallow bowl. Add the haloumi slices and toss to coat. Place the haloumi slices on a grill rack lined with foil and cook under a preheated hot grill for 2-3 minutes until browned in places.

4   Stir the couscous into the chickpea mixture and cook for 1 minute to heat through. Serve the couscous piled on to serving plates, topped with the grilled haloumi slices.

200 g (7 oz) couscous
5 tablespoons olive oil
2 red onions, thinly sliced
1 red chilli, roughly chopped
400 g (13 oz) can chickpeas, rinsed and drained
175 g (6 oz) cherry tomatoes, halved
3 tablespoons chopped parsley
1 tablespoon finely chopped thyme leaves
375 g (12 oz) haloumi cheese, thickly sliced
salt

Serves **4**
Prep time **15 minutes, plus soaking**
Cooking time **10 minutes**

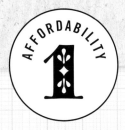

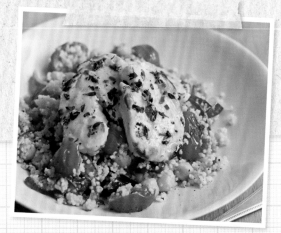

Lentil Moussaka (V)

1 Put the lentils in a saucepan with the tomatoes, garlic, oregano and nutmeg. Pour in the stock. Bring to the boil, then reduce the heat and simmer for 20 minutes until the lentils are tender but not mushy, topping up with extra stock as needed.

2 Meanwhile, heat the oil in a frying pan and lightly fry the aubergine slices and onion until the onion is soft and the aubergine is golden on both sides.

3 Layer the aubergine mixture and lentil mixture alternately in an ovenproof dish.

4 Make the topping. In a bowl, beat together the egg, soft cheese and nutmeg with a good dash of salt and pepper. Pour over the moussaka and cook in a preheated oven, 200°C (400°F), Gas Mark 6, for 20-25 minutes or until golden and bubbling. Remove from the oven and leave to stand for 5 minutes before serving with a mixed leaf salad.

VARIATION

For moussaka baked potatoes, bake 4 scrubbed baking potatoes, about 200 g (7 oz) each, in a preheated oven, 200°C (400°F), Gas Mark 6, for about 1 hour until cooked and tender (or microwave them, if preferred). Meanwhile, make the lentil mixture as above. Fry the aubergine slices and onion separately, then stir into the lentils when cooked. Spoon over the slit potatoes, then top each one with a spoonful of soft cheese and a sprinkling of grated Cheddar-style cheese.

125 g (4 oz) brown or green lentils, rinsed and drained
400 g (13 oz) can chopped tomatoes
2 garlic cloves, crushed
½ teaspoon dried oregano
pinch of ground (or freshly grated) nutmeg
150 ml (¼ pint) Vegetable Stock (see page 244)
2-3 tablespoons vegetable oil
250 g (8 oz) aubergines, sliced
1 onion, finely chopped
mixed leaf salad, to serve

Cheese topping
1 egg
150 g (5 oz) soft cheese
pinch of ground (or freshly grated) nutmeg
salt and pepper

Serves **4**
Prep time **10 minutes**
Cooking time **45 minutes, plus standing**

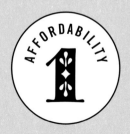

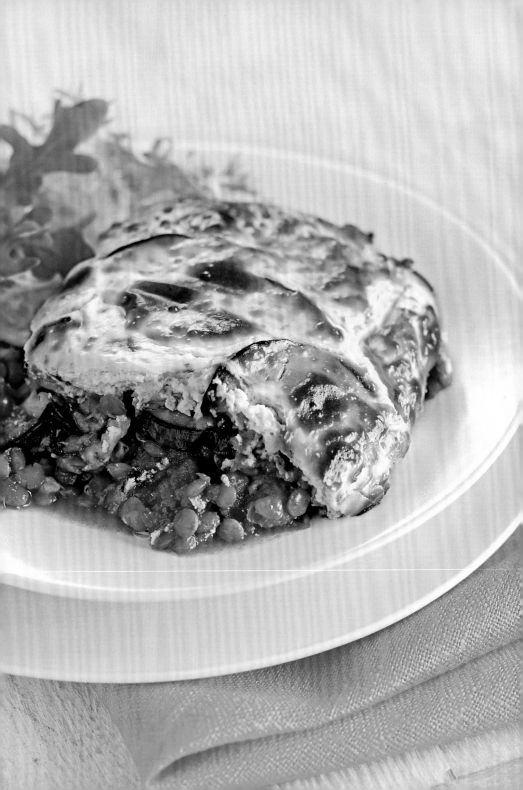

LAYERED LENTIL & QUINOA
NUT ROAST

1. Cook the quinoa in a saucepan of boiling water for 15-20 minutes or until tender. Drain thoroughly and transfer to a bowl.

2. Heat the oil in a separate saucepan and fry the onion for 5 minutes to soften. Slide half of the mixture out into the bowl of quinoa. Add the celery to the pan and fry for 2 minutes. Stir in the spice, lentils and stock and bring to the boil. Reduce the heat to a gentle simmer and cook, uncovered, for 10 minutes or until the mixture is dry and the lentils are tender. Remove from the heat, stir in the dates and leave to cool.

3. Crumble the almonds into the quinoa. Beat in the coriander, whole egg and a little salt and pepper. Beat the egg yolk into the cooled lentil mixture.

4. Oil a 500 g (1 lb) loaf tin and line the base and long sides with strips of nonstick baking paper.

5. Spoon half of the quinoa mixture into the prepared tin and press down firmly. Spoon half of the lentil mixture on top and level the surface. Add the remaining quinoa and lentil mixtures, spreading them evenly.

6. Bake in a preheated oven 180°C (350°F), Gas Mark 4, for 30 minutes until the loaf feels firm. Turn out on to a board and serve in slices.

100 g (3½ oz) quinoa, rinsed and drained
1 tablespoon olive oil, plus extra for greasing
1 onion, finely chopped
1 celery stick, chopped
2 teaspoons ras el hanout spice
100 g (3½ oz) split red lentils, rinsed and drained
300 ml (½ pint) Vegetable Stock (see page 244)
25 g (1 oz) pitted dried dates, finely chopped
50 g (2 oz) flaked almonds
2 tablespoons finely chopped fresh coriander
1 egg, beaten
1 egg yolk
salt and pepper

Serves **8**
Prep time **25 minutes, plus cooling**
Cooking time **1 hour 10 minutes**

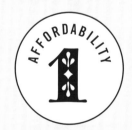

HOME-BAKED BEANS

THESE HOME-BAKED BEANS ARE EVEN BETTER MADE A DAY AHEAD, THEN KEPT REFRIGERATED OVERNIGHT AND HEATED THROUGH UNTIL PIPING HOT BEFORE SERVING.

1 Put all the ingredients in a flameproof casserole with a little salt and pepper. Cover and bring slowly to the boil.

2 Transfer to a preheated oven, 160°C (325°F), Gas Mark 3, and bake for 1½ hours. Remove the lid, stir, then bake for a further 30 minutes until the sauce is syrupy. Serve with hot buttered toast, if liked.

VARIATION

For home-baked beans with baked potatoes, scrub 4 baking potatoes, about 200 g (7 oz) each, then bake in a preheated oven, 200°C (400°F), Gas Mark 6, for about 1 hour until cooked and tender (or microwave them, if preferred). Cut the potatoes in half lengthways, season with salt and pepper and then spoon over the home-baked beans. Grate over a little Cheddar-style cheese before serving.

2 x 400 g (13 oz) cans borlotti beans, rinsed and drained
1 garlic clove, crushed
1 onion, finely chopped
450 ml (¾ pint) Vegetable Stock (see page 244)
300 ml (½ pint) passata (sieved tomatoes)
2 tablespoons molasses or black treacle
2 tablespoons tomato purée
2 tablespoons soft dark brown sugar
1 tablespoon Dijon mustard
1 tablespoon red wine vinegar
salt and pepper
hot buttered toast, to serve (optional)

Serves **4**
Prep time **10 minutes**
Cooking time **2 hours 10 minutes**

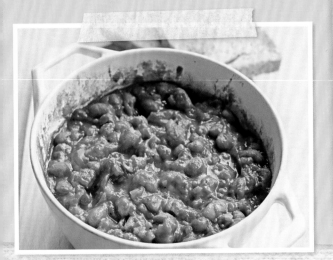

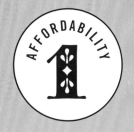
AFFORDABILITY
1

ROASTED ROOTS
and quinoa salad ♥ Vegan

1 Put the beetroot and carrots in a roasting tin. Drizzle over the olive oil, sprinkle with the cumin seeds and season well with salt and pepper, then toss until the roots are evenly coated in the oil. Roast in a preheated oven, 200°C (400°F), Gas Mark 6, for 30–35 minutes until tender.

2 Meanwhile, cook the quinoa in a saucepan of boiling water for 10–12 minutes until tender, then drain. Tip into a large bowl, add the chickpeas, onion, mint and hazelnuts and toss together.

3 Mix the lime juice, tamari or soy sauce and sesame oil together in a jug, pour over the quinoa mixture and gently toss together. Add the roasted beetroots and carrots and lightly mix through, then serve.

VARIATION

For roasted carrot and parsnip salad with edamame (soya) beans, toss 300 g (10 oz) each of scrubbed baby carrots and baby parsnips with 1 tablespoon olive oil, 1 teaspoon cumin seeds and salt and pepper in a roasting tin. Roast in a preheated oven, 200°C (400°F), Gas Mark 6, for 20–25 minutes until tender. Meanwhile, cook the quinoa as above, adding 125 g (4 oz) frozen edamame (soya) beans for the final 3 minutes of the cooking time. Drain and tip into a large bowl. Add 1 thinly sliced red onion, a handful of roughly chopped flat leaf parsley and 2 tablespoons toasted blanched almonds, roughly chopped. Make the lime juice dressing as above, pour over the quinoa mixture and gently toss together. Add the roasted carrots and parsnips and lightly mix through.

300 g (10 oz) raw baby beetroot, scrubbed and halved or quartered if large
300 g (10 oz) baby carrots, scrubbed
1 tablespoon olive oil
1 teaspoon cumin seeds
150 g (5 oz) quinoa, rinsed and drained
400 g (13 oz) can chickpeas, rinsed and drained
1 small red onion, thinly sliced
small handful of mint leaves, roughly chopped
2 tablespoons blanched hazelnuts, roughly chopped
juice of 1 lime
1 tablespoon tamari or soy sauce
1 teaspoon sesame oil
salt and pepper

Serves **4**
Prep time **10 minutes**
Cooking time **30-35 minutes**

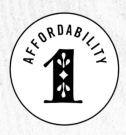
AFFORDABILITY 1

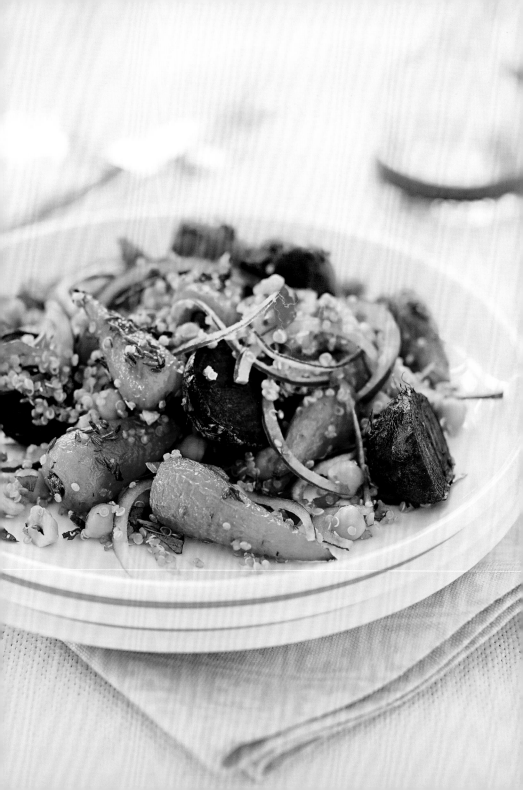

Super Salads, Snacks & Sides

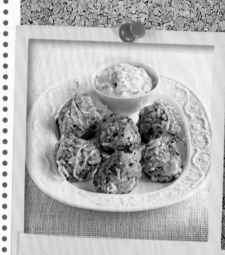

SALMON & RICE BHAJIS

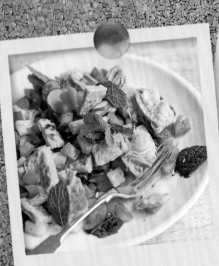

FATTOUSH SALAD

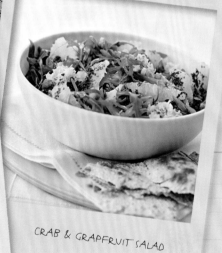

CRAB & GRAPFRUIT SALAD

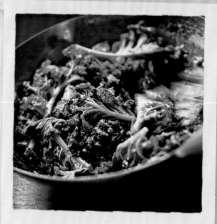

CHILLI KALE

COCONUT NOODLES IN A MUG

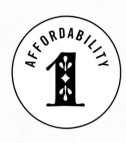

1 Mix together the spring onions, courgette and oil in a large, microwave-proof mug and microwave on medium power for 2 minutes.

2 Stir in the coconut milk, bouillon powder, Thai spice, turmeric, if using, and the boiling water. Microwave on medium power for 1 minute.

3 Break the noodles into the mug and stir to mix. Microwave on medium power for 1 minute. Stir again and microwave on medium power for a further 1½ minutes until the noodles are tender. Sprinkle with the cashew nuts and serve.

3 spring onions, thinly sliced
100 g (3½ oz) courgette, grated
1 teaspoon wok oil
100 ml (3½ fl oz) coconut milk
¼ teaspoon vegetable bouillon powder
½ teaspoon Thai spice powder, such as Thai 7 spice or Thai 5 spice
good pinch of ground turmeric (optional)
75 ml (3 fl oz) boiling water
25 g (1 oz) vermicelli rice noodles
10 cashew nuts, roughly chopped

Makes **1**
Prep time **5 minutes**
Cooking time **5½ minutes**

MASSAMAN LENTILS
with Cauliflower

1. Cook the lentils in a saucepan of boiling water for 15 minutes until softened but not falling apart. Drain well.

2. Meanwhile, melt the butter with the oil in a separate saucepan. Add the onions and carrot and fry gently for 5 minutes, stirring frequently. Add the cauliflower and fry for a further 5 minutes.

3. Stir in the curry paste, sugar, ginger and stock and bring to a gentle simmer. Cook very gently, stirring frequently, for 10 minutes until the cauliflower is tender.

4. Stir in the lentils and basil, season to taste with salt and pepper and then serve with boiled jasmine or long-grain rice.

150 g (5 oz) green lentils, rinsed and drained
20 g (¾ oz) butter
1 teaspoon oil
2 onions, sliced
1 large carrot, thinly sliced
1 small cauliflower or ½ large cauliflower, about 400 g (13 oz), cut into large florets
1 tablespoon Massaman curry paste
1 teaspoon light muscovado or caster sugar
1.5 cm (¾ inch) piece of fresh root ginger, peeled and grated
500 ml (17 fl oz) Vegetable Stock (see page 244)
small handful of Thai basil, torn into pieces
salt and pepper
Boiled Rice (see page 247), to serve

Serves **2**
Prep time **10 minutes**
Cooking time **20 minutes**

AFFORDABILITY
1

QUICK CURRIED EGG SALAD

1 Shell, then halve the eggs and place on a large platter with the tomatoes, lettuce leaves and cucumber.

2 Mix the yogurt with the curry powder, tomato purée, lime juice and mayonnaise in a small bowl. Season the dressing with salt and pepper to taste, then pour it over the salad. Serve immediately, garnished with thyme leaves.

8 hard-boiled eggs
4 tomatoes, cut into wedges
2 Little Gem lettuces, leaves separated
½ cucumber, sliced
200 ml (7 fl oz) natural yogurt
1 tablespoon mild curry powder
3 tablespoons tomato purée
juice of 2 limes
6 tablespoons mayonnaise
salt and pepper
thyme leaves, to garnish

Serves **4**
Prep time **10 minutes**

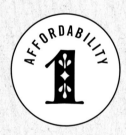

HEALTHY TIP

SNACK ATTACK Keep a cereal bar, piece of fresh fruit, some dried fruit or a snack bag of unsalted nuts or seeds in your bag for when you have a sudden energy slump. If there's a healthy snack on tap, you'll be less likely to raid the canteen for a doughnut (see page 74 for healthy snack ideas).

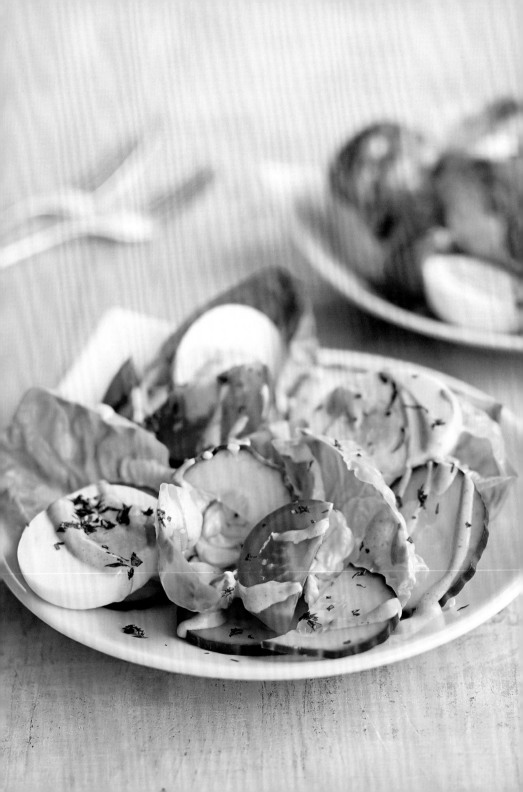

ROASTED VEGETABLE COUSCOUS SALAD

1 Place all the vegetables on a large nonstick baking tray in a single layer. Drizzle with a little oil and season well with salt and pepper. Roast in a preheated oven, 200°C (400°F), Gas Mark 6, for 15-20 minutes or until the edges of the vegetables are just starting to char.

2 Meanwhile, put the couscous in a wide bowl and pour over enough boiling water to just cover. Season well. Cover with clingfilm and leave to stand, undisturbed, for 10 minutes or until all the liquid has been absorbed. Fluff up the grains with a fork and place on a wide, shallow serving platter.

3 Make the dressing by mixing together the orange juice, oil, cumin and cinnamon and season well with salt and pepper.

4 Fold the roasted vegetables, preserved lemons and herbs into the couscous, pour over the dressing and toss to mix well.

5 Scatter over the pine nuts, feta and pomegranate seeds and serve immediately.

1 red pepper, deseeded and cut into 2.5 cm (1 inch) pieces
1 yellow pepper, deseeded and cut into 2.5 cm (1 inch) pieces
1 medium aubergine, cut into 2.5 cm (1 inch) pieces
1 courgette, cut into 2.5 cm (1 inch) cubes
2 small red onions, cut into thick wedges
olive oil, to drizzle
200 g (7 oz) couscous
6-8 preserved lemons, halved
large handful of mint and coriander leaves, chopped
50 g (2 oz) pine nuts, toasted
150 g (5 oz) feta cheese, crumbled
100 g (3½ oz) pomegranate seeds
salt and pepper

Dressing
juice of 1 orange
5 tablespoons olive oil
1 teaspoon ground cumin
1 teaspoon ground cinnamon

Serves **4**
Prep time **15 minutes**
Cooking time **15-20 minutes**

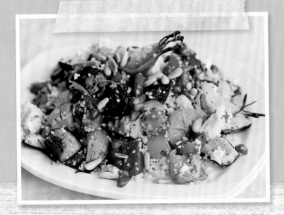

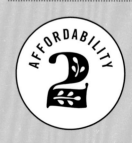

AFFORDABILITY 2

FATTOUSH SALAD

1. First make the dressing. Whisk the oil, lemon juice, garlic and sumac or cumin together in a bowl. Season to taste with salt and pepper.

2. To make the salad, combine the pitta pieces, tomatoes, cucumber, radishes, onion, lettuce leaves and mint leaves in a large bowl.

3. Pour the dressing over the salad and gently mix together to coat the salad evenly.

1 pitta bread, torn into small pieces
6 plum tomatoes, deseeded and roughly chopped
1 cucumber, peeled and roughly chopped
10 radishes, sliced
1 red onion, roughly chopped
1 small Little Gem lettuce, leaves separated
small handful of fresh mint leaves

Dressing

200 ml (7 fl oz) olive oil
juice of 3 lemons
1 garlic clove, crushed
2 teaspoons sumac or 2 teaspoons ground cumin
salt and pepper

Serves **4**
Prep time **15 minutes**

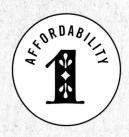

AFFORDABILITY 1

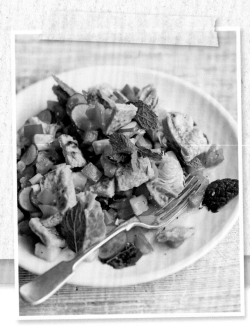

Tricolore Avocado & Couscous Salad (V)

1 Mix the couscous and stock or boiling water together in a bowl, then cover with clingfilm and leave to stand for 10 minutes.

2 Meanwhile, to make the dressing, mix the pesto with the lemon juice in a small bowl. Season with salt and pepper, then gradually mix in the oil.

3 Pour the dressing over the couscous and mix with a fork. Add the tomatoes, avocados and mozzarella to the couscous, mix well, then lightly stir in the rocket. Serve.

200 g (7 oz) couscous
300 ml (½ pint) hot Vegetable Stock (see page 244) or boiling water
250 g (8 oz) cherry tomatoes
2 ripe avocados, peeled, stoned and chopped
150 g (5 oz) mozzarella cheese, drained and chopped
handful of rocket

Dressing
2 tablespoons Pesto (see page 248)
1 tablespoon lemon juice
4 tablespoons extra virgin olive oil
salt and pepper

Serves **4**
Prep time **20 minutes**

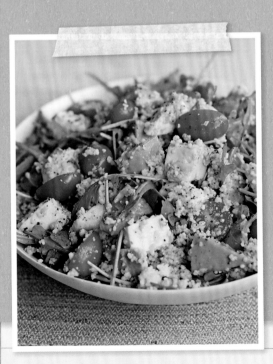

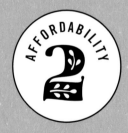

AFFORDABILITY 2

Italian
BROCCOLI & EGG SALAD

1 Put the broccoli in the top of a steamer, cook for 3 minutes, then add the leeks and cook for a further 2 minutes.

2 Mix together the lemon juice, oil, honey, capers and chopped tarragon in a salad bowl and season to taste with salt and pepper. Shell and roughly chop the eggs.

3 Add the broccoli and leeks to the dressing, toss together and then sprinkle with the chopped eggs. Garnish with tarragon sprigs and serve warm with extra-thick slices of wholemeal bread, if liked.

VARIATION
For a broccoli, cauliflower and egg salad, use 150 g (5 oz) broccoli and 150 g (5 oz) cauliflower instead of 300 g (10 oz) broccoli. Cut the cauliflower into small florets and steam with the broccoli. Serve with a blue cheese dressing made by mixing together 75 g (3 oz) blue cheese, 6 chopped sun-dried tomatoes and 3 tablespoons balsamic vinegar.

300 g (10 oz) broccoli, cut into florets and stems thickly sliced
2 small leeks, about 300 g (10 oz) in total, trimmed, cleaned and thickly sliced
4 tablespoons lemon juice
2 tablespoons olive oil
2 teaspoons clear honey
1 tablespoon capers, drained
2 tablespoons chopped tarragon, plus extra sprigs to garnish
4 hard-boiled eggs
salt and pepper
extra-thick slices of wholemeal bread, to serve (optional)

Serves **4**
Prep time **15 minutes**
Cooking time **5 minutes**

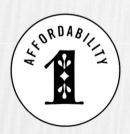

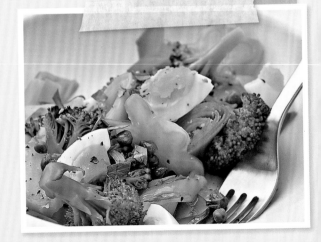

GREEK SALAD
WITH TOASTED PITTA (V)

1 Put the feta, mint, olives, tomatoes, lemon juice, onion and oregano in a bowl and toss together to mix.

2 Toast the pitta breads under a preheated hot grill until lightly golden, turning once, then split open and toast the open sides.

3 Tear the hot pittas into bite-sized pieces, then toss with the other ingredients in the bowl. Serve immediately with lemon wedges.

100 g (3½ oz) feta cheese, crumbled into smallish chunks
8-10 fresh mint leaves, shredded
100 g (3½ oz) kalamata olives, pitted
2 tomatoes, chopped
juice of 1 large lemon
1 small red onion, thinly sliced
1 teaspoon dried oregano
4 pitta breads
lemon wedges, to serve

Serves **4**
Prep time **15 minutes**
Cooking time **5 minutes**

HEALTHY TIP

SWITCH REGULAR FIZZY DRINKS FOR LOW-CALORIE VERSIONS

Carbonated drinks aren't exactly a healthy addition to your diet but if you're going to treat yourself, at least make it sugar-free.

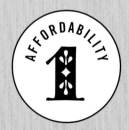

AFFORDABILITY 1

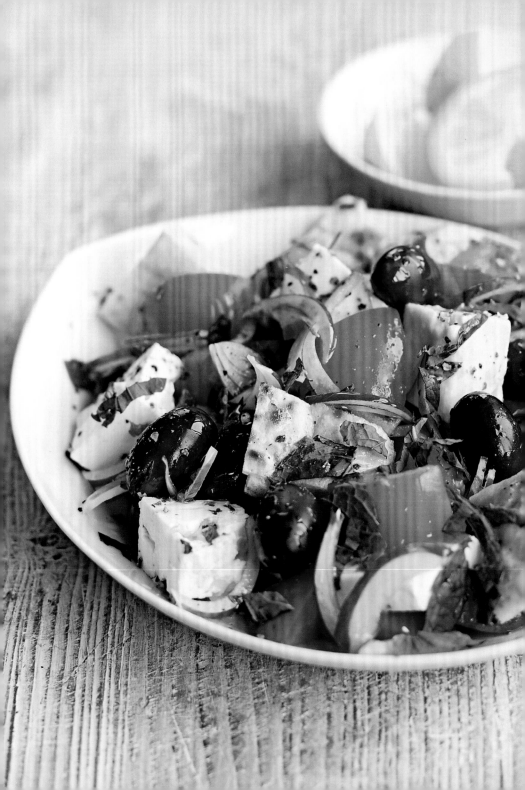

SMOKED MACKEREL SUPERFOOD SALAD

1 Place the squash in a roasting tin and sprinkle with 1 tablespoon of the oil and the cumin seeds. Place in a preheated oven, 200°C (400°F), Gas Mark 6, for 15-18 minutes until tender. Leave to cool slightly.

2 Meanwhile, cook the broccoli in a saucepan of boiling water for 4-5 minutes until tender, adding the peas 3 minutes before the end of the cooking time. Remove with a slotted spoon and refresh under cold running water, then drain (reserving the cooking water). Cook the quinoa in the broccoli water for 15 minutes, then drain and leave to cool slightly.

3 Heat a nonstick frying pan over a medium-low heat and dry-fry the seeds, stirring frequently, until golden brown and toasted. Set aside. Heat the mackerel fillets according to the packet instructions, then skin and break into flakes.

4 Whisk together the remaining oil, the lemon juice, honey and mustard in a small bowl. Toss together all the ingredients, except the radish sprouts, with the dressing in a serving bowl. Serve topped with the radish sprouts.

500 g (1 lb) butternut squash, peeled, deseeded and cut into 1 cm (½ inch) cubes
4 tablespoons olive oil
1 teaspoon cumin seeds
1 head of broccoli, cut into florets
200 g (7 oz) frozen or fresh peas
3 tablespoons quinoa, rinsed and drained
4 tablespoons mixed seeds
2 smoked mackerel fillets
juice of 1 lemon
1 teaspoon clear honey
1 Dijon mustard
100 g (3⅓ oz) red cabbage, shredded
4 tomatoes, chopped
4 cooked beetroot, cut into wedges
20 g (¾ oz) radish sprouts

Serves **4**
Prep time **20 minutes**
Cooking time **25-30 minutes**

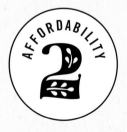

COURGETTE, FETA & MINT SALAD

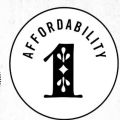

1. Thinly slice the courgettes lengthways into long ribbons. Drizzle with oil and season with salt and pepper. Heat a griddle pan until it's very hot, then grill the courgettes, in batches, until tender and griddle-marked on both sides. Transfer to a large salad bowl.

2. Make the dressing by whisking together the oil and lemon rind and juice in a small bowl. Season to taste with salt and pepper.

3. Roughly chop the mint, reserving some leaves for the garnish. Carefully mix together the griddled courgettes, chopped mint and dressing in the salad bowl, then crumble the feta over the top, garnish with the remaining mint leaves and serve.

VARIATION
For marinated courgette salad, thinly slice 3 courgettes lengthways and put them in a non-metallic bowl with ½ deseeded and sliced red chilli, 4 tablespoons lemon juice, 1 crushed garlic clove and 4 tablespoons olive oil. Season to taste with salt and pepper. Leave the salad to marinate, covered, for at least 1 hour. Roughly chop a small bunch of mint leaves, toss with the salad and serve immediately.

3 green courgettes
2 yellow courgettes
olive oil, for drizzling
small bunch of mint leaves
40 g (1½ oz) feta cheese
salt and pepper

Dressing
2 tablespoons olive oil
finely grated rind and juice of
  1 lemon

Serves **4**
Prep time **15 minutes**
Cooking time **10 minutes**

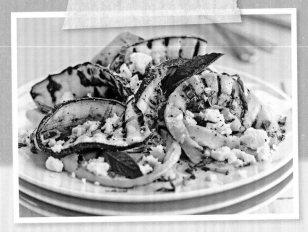

BRAINFOOD BOWL (V)

1 Cook the rice in a large saucepan of lightly salted water for 25 minutes or until just tender.

2 Meanwhile, cut the broccoli into smaller pieces and cook in a separate saucepan of boiling water for 2 minutes until softened. Add the sugar snap peas and cook for a further 30 seconds. Drain, rinse under cold running water, then drain again.

3 Lightly toast the hazelnuts in a dry frying pan, shaking the pan frequently until the nuts start to colour. Add the pumpkin seeds and cook for a further 1-2 minutes until they start to pop.

4 Thoroughly drain the rice and mix in a bowl with the broccoli, sugar snap peas, nuts and seeds.

5 Halve the grapefruit. Squeeze the juice from one half into a small bowl. Cut away the skin and white pith from the remaining half and chop the flesh. Add to the rice bowl. Peel, halve, stone and dice the avocado and add to the grapefruit juice. Toss to coat, then lift out with a slotted spoon and add to the rice.

6 Whisk the ginger, oil and honey into the grapefruit juice. Stir the dressing into the rice mixture just before serving. Season to taste with salt and pepper and serve.

100 g (3 ½ oz) brown rice
150 g (5 oz) broccoli florets
75 g (3 oz) sugar snap peas, halved lengthways
50 g (2 oz) hazelnuts, roughly chopped
25 g (1 oz) pumpkin seeds
1 pink or red grapefruit
1 ripe avocado
25 g (1 oz) fresh root ginger, peeled and grated
1 tablespoon olive oil
1 tablespoon clear honey
salt and pepper

Serves **2**
Prep time **20 minutes**
Cooking time **25 minutes**

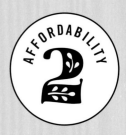

AFFORDABILITY 2

SOY TOFU SALAD
WITH CORIANDER

1 Cut the tofu into bite-sized cubes and carefully arrange on a serving plate in a single layer. Sprinkle over the spring onions, coriander and chilli.

2 Drizzle over the soy sauce and oil, then leave to stand at room temperature for 10 minutes before serving.

VARIATION

For steamed chilli-soy tofu, drain 500 g (1 lb) firm tofu, cut it into bite-sized cubes and place it on a heatproof plate that will fit inside a bamboo steamer. Cover and steam over a wok or large saucepan of boiling water for 20 minutes, then drain off the excess water and carefully transfer to a serving plate. Heat 4 tablespoons light soy sauce, 1 tablespoon each sesame oil and groundnut oil and 2 teaspoons oyster sauce in a small saucepan until hot. Pour over the tofu, scatter with 4 thinly sliced spring onions, 1 finely chopped red chilli and a small handful of finely chopped fresh coriander leaves and serve.

500 g (1 lb) firm tofu, drained
6 spring onions, finely shredded
large handful of fresh coriander
   leaves, roughly chopped
1 large mild red chilli, deseeded
   and thinly sliced
4 tablespoons light soy sauce
2 teaspoons sesame oil

Serves **4**
Prep time **10 minutes,
plus standing**

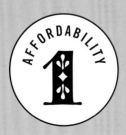

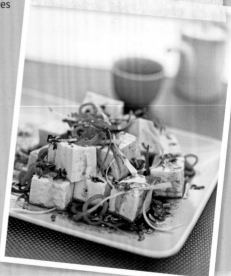

SPICED CHICKEN & MANGO SALAD

1 Put 4 teaspoons of the curry paste into a polythene food bag with the lemon juice and mix together by squeezing the bag. Add the chicken pieces and toss together.

2 Half-fill the base of a steamer with water and bring to the boil. Remove the chicken from the bag and place in the top of the steamer in a single layer. Cover and steam for 5-6 minutes until cooked through.

3 Meanwhile, mix the remaining curry paste in a bowl with the yogurt. Put the mango, watercress, cucumber and onion in a bowl, add the yogurt dressing and toss together gently.

4 Tear the lettuce into pieces, divide it between 4 plates, then spoon the mango mixture on top. Add the warm chicken strips on top, then serve.

VARIATION

For coronation chicken, mix the curry paste and yogurt with 4 tablespoons reduced-fat mayonnaise. Stir in 500 g (1 lb) cold cooked diced chicken and 40 g (1½ oz) sultanas. Sprinkle with 25 g (1 oz) toasted flaked almonds and serve on a bed of mixed salad and herb leaves.

6 teaspoons mild curry paste
juice of 1 lemon
4 small boneless, skinless chicken breasts, cut into long, thin strips
150 g (5 oz) natural yogurt
1 ripe mango, peeled, stoned and cut into bite-sized chunks
50 g (2 oz) watercress, torn into smaller pieces
½ cucumber, diced
½ red onion, chopped
½ iceberg lettuce

Serves **4**
Prep time **5 minutes**
Cooking time **5-6 minutes**

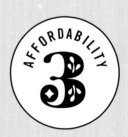

AFFORDABILITY

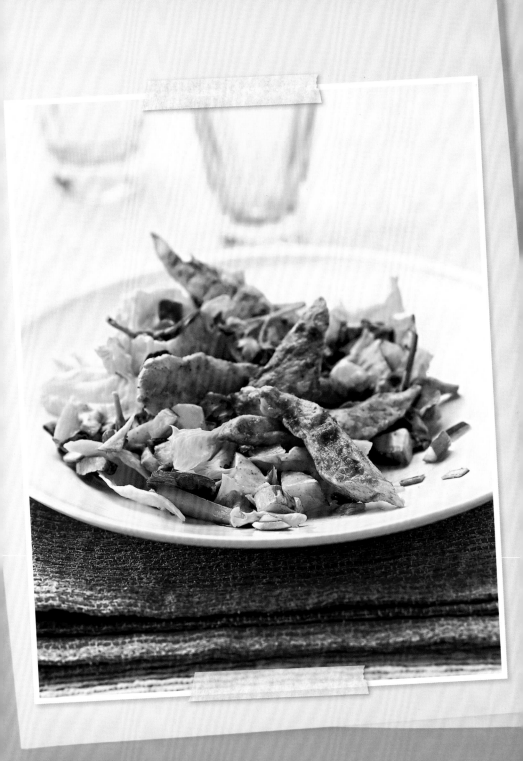

TANDOORI CHICKEN SALAD

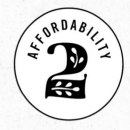

1 Mix the yogurt, lemon juice, spices, tomato purée, garlic and ginger together in a shallow, non-metallic dish. Add the chicken and toss to coat. Cover and leave to marinate in the refrigerator for 3–4 hours or until required.

2 When you are ready to serve, heat the oil in a large frying pan. Lift the chicken out of the marinade and add to the pan. Cook over a medium heat for 8–10 minutes, turning occasionally, until the chicken is browned and cooked through.

3 Meanwhile, for the salad, toss the salad leaves, coriander and lemon juice together in a bowl and then divide between serving plates. Spoon the hot chicken on top and serve immediately.

VARIATION
For tandoori chicken skewers, thread 350 g (12 oz) diced boneless, skinless chicken breasts on to 8 pre-soaked wooden skewers. Place in a large, shallow, non-metallic dish, then spoon over the yogurt marinade and chill as above. When you are ready to serve, lift the kebabs out of the marinade and cook under a preheated hot grill, turning occasionally, until the chicken is cooked through. Serve with the salad dressed with lemon juice as above.

200 ml (7 fl oz) natural yogurt
2 tablespoons lemon juice
½ teaspoon ground turmeric
1 teaspoon garam masala
1 teaspoon cumin seeds, roughly crushed
2 tablespoons tomato purée
2 garlic cloves, finely chopped
1.5 cm (¾ inch) piece of fresh root ginger, peeled and finely chopped
3 boneless, skinless chicken breasts, thickly sliced
1 tablespoon sunflower oil

Salad
200 g (7 oz) mixed salad leaves
small bunch of fresh coriander
4 tablespoons lemon juice

Serves **4**
Prep time **15 minutes, plus marinating**
Cooking time **10 minutes**

TURKEY & AVOCADO SALAD

1 large ripe avocado, peeled,
  stoned and diced
1 punnet of mustard and cress, cut
150 g (5 oz) mixed salad leaves
375 g (12 oz) cooked turkey, thinly
  sliced
50 g (2 oz) mixed toasted seeds,
  such as pumpkin and sunflower
toasted wholegrain rye bread or
  flatbreads, to serve

Dressing
2 tablespoons apple juice
2 tablespoons natural yogurt
1 teaspoon clear honey
1 teaspoon wholegrain mustard
salt and pepper

Serves **4**
Prep time **15 minutes**

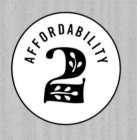

1 Put the avocado, mustard and cress and salad leaves in a large bowl and mix together. Add the turkey and toasted seeds and stir to combine.

2 Make the dressing by whisking together the apple juice, yogurt, honey and mustard in a small bowl. Season to taste with salt and pepper.

3 Pour the dressing over the salad and toss to mix. Serve the salad with toasted wholegrain rye bread or rolled up in flatbreads.

VARIATION
For a crab, apple and avocado salad, prepare the salad in the same way, using 300 g (10 oz) cooked, fresh white crab meat instead of the turkey. Cut 1 peeled and cored dessert apple into thin matchsticks and toss with a little lemon juice to stop it from discolouring. Add to the crab salad. Make a dressing by whisking together 2 tablespoons apple juice, 3 tablespoons olive oil, a squeeze of lemon juice and 1 finely diced shallot. Season to taste with salt and pepper. Pour the dressing over the salad, stir carefully to mix and serve.

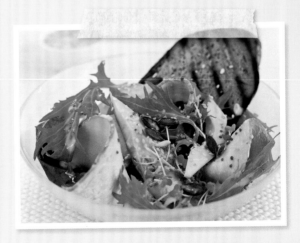

TUNA & BORLOTTI BEAN SALAD

1 Heat the borlotti beans in a saucepan over a medium heat for 3 minutes, adding the water if the beans start to stick to the base.

2 Put the oil, garlic and chilli in a large bowl. Stir in the celery, onion and hot beans and season with salt and pepper. Cover and leave to marinate at room temperature for at least 30 minutes and up to 4 hours.

3 Stir in the tuna and lemon rind and juice. Gently toss in the rocket, taste and adjust the seasoning with extra salt, pepper and lemon juice, if necessary, then serve.

VARIATION

For a mixed bean salad, heat the borlotti beans, as above, with a 400 g (13 oz) can rinsed and drained cannellini beans. Leave to marinate with the other salad ingredients as above, but also adding 2 tablespoons roughly chopped flat leaf parsley. After marinating, toss in 50 g (2 oz) lamb's lettuce, season with salt and pepper and serve.

400 g (13 oz) can borlotti beans, rinsed and drained
1 tablespoon water (optional)
2 tablespoons extra virgin olive oil
2 garlic cloves, crushed
1 red chilli, deseeded and finely chopped
2 celery sticks, thinly sliced
½ red onion, cut into thin wedges
200 g (7 oz) can tuna in olive oil, drained and flaked
finely grated rind and juice of 1 lemon
50 g (2 oz) rocket leaves
salt and pepper

Serves **4**
Prep time **15 minutes, plus marinating**
Cooking time **3 minutes**

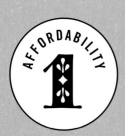

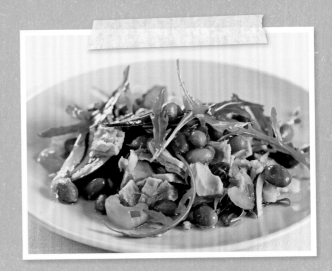

Crab & Grapefruit

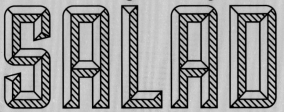
SALAD

1 Combine the crab meat, grapefruit, rocket, spring onions and mangetout in a serving dish. Season to taste with salt and pepper.

2 Make the dressing by whisking together the watercress, mustard and oil in a small bowl. Season to taste with salt.

3 Toast the chapattis. Stir the dressing into the crab salad, then serve with the toasted chapattis and lime wedges on the side.

VARIATION
For a prawn, potato and asparagus salad, substitute 400 g (13 oz) cooked peeled prawns for the crab and 100 g (3½ oz) cooked asparagus for the grapefruit, and add 200 g (7 oz) cooked and cooled potatoes.

400 g (13 oz) white crab meat
1 pink grapefruit, peeled, white pith removed and flesh sliced
50 g (2 oz) rocket
3 spring onions, sliced
200 g (7 oz) mangetout, halved
salt and pepper

Watercress dressing
90 g (3 ¼ oz) watercress (tough stalks removed), chopped
1 tablespoon Dijon mustard
2 tablespoons olive oil

To serve
4 chapattis
lime wedges

Serves **4**
Prep time **15 minutes**

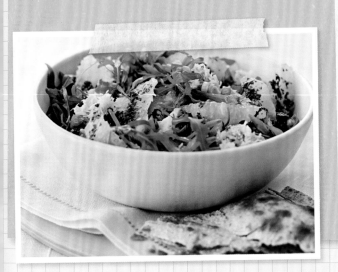

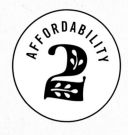

AFFORDABILITY 2

QUICK ONE-POT RATATOUILLE

Vegan

1 Heat the oil in a large saucepan until very hot. Add the onions, aubergine, courgettes, peppers and garlic and cook, stirring constantly, for a few minutes until softened.

2 Add the tomatoes, season with salt and pepper and stir well. Reduce the heat, cover the pan tightly and simmer for 15 minutes until all the vegetables are cooked. Remove from the heat and stir in the parsley or basil before serving.

100 ml (3½ fl oz) olive oil
2 onions, chopped
1 aubergine, cut into bite-sized cubes
2 large courgettes, cut into bite-sized pieces
1 red pepper, cored, deseeded and cut into bite-sized pieces
1 yellow pepper, cored, deseeded and cut into bite-sized pieces
2 garlic cloves, crushed
400 g (13 oz) can chopped tomatoes
4 tablespoons chopped parsley or basil
salt and pepper

Serves **4**
Prep time **10 minutes**
Cooking time **20 minutes**

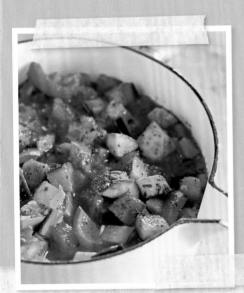

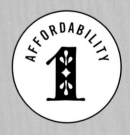

AFFORDABILITY
1

GOATS' CHEESE & SPINACH
QUESADILLAS

1 Place the spinach in a saucepan with a small amount of water, then cover and cook until wilted. Drain and squeeze dry.

2 Heat a nonstick frying pan over medium heat until hot, add 1 tortilla and then crumble a quarter of the goats' cheese, followed by a quarter of the spinach and sun-dried tomatoes, over the tortilla. Season lightly with salt and pepper.

3 Place 1 tortilla on top and cook for 3–4 minutes until golden underneath. Carefully turn the quesadilla over and cook for a further 3–4 minutes. Remove from the pan and keep warm. Repeat with the remaining 6 tortillas.

4 Meanwhile, mix together the avocados, onion, lime juice and coriander in a bowl.

5 Serve the warm quesadillas cut into wedges with the avocado salsa.

275 g (9 oz) baby spinach leaves
8 soft flour tortillas
250 g (8 oz) goats' cheese
2 tablespoons drained, chopped sun-dried tomatoes
2 ripe avocados, peeled, stoned and diced
1 red onion, thinly sliced
juice of 1 lime
2 tablespoons chopped fresh coriander
salt and pepper

Serves **4**
Prep time **10 minutes**
Cooking time **25-35 minutes**

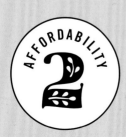

AFFORDABILITY
2

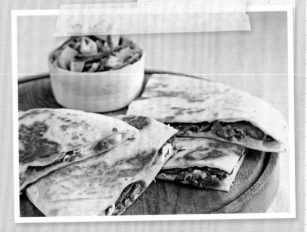

SMOKED MACKEREL & CHIVE PÂTÉ

1 Place the mackerel and soft cheese in a bowl and mash together well. Add all the remaining ingredients and mix well. Alternatively, mix all the ingredients together in a blender or food processor.

2 Spoon the mixture into 8 small individual serving dishes or 1 large serving dish. Cover and refrigerate for at least 2 hours or up to 4 hours, before serving.

3 Serve the mackerel pâté with vegetable crudités and wholemeal toast, if liked.

VARIATION
Try using other omega-3-rich fish instead of mackerel in this recipe, such as canned (in water) drained pilchards, salmon or tuna.

1200 g (7 oz) smoked mackerel, skinned, boned and flaked
125 g (4 oz) low-fat soft cheese
bunch of chives, snipped
1 tablespoon fat-free vinaigrette
1 tablespoon lemon juice
vegetable crudités and wholemeal toast, to serve (optional)

Serves **8**
Prep time **10 minutes, plus chilling**

HEALTHY TIP
Of all the oily fish that are readily available, mackerel is the richest source of omega-3 fatty acids, so enjoy it in all its many forms — fresh, canned or smoked. It is also one of the least expensive oily fish.

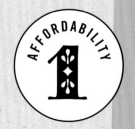

HOT & SMOKY HUMMUS WITH WARM FLATBREAD

 Vegan

LEBANESE FLATBREAD IS A ROUND, FLAT, SLIGHTLY PUFFY BREAD, WHICH GOES VERY WELL WITH MEZZE DIPS. IF YOU CAN'T GET HOLD OF IT, PITTAS OR EVEN SOFT FLOUR TORTILLAS WOULD MAKE A GOOD SUBSTITUTE.

1 Put all the ingredients, except the olive oil and sesame seeds, in a blender or food processor and process until smooth. With the machine still running, very slowly drizzle the oil into the chickpea paste until it is all completely incorporated. Season to taste with salt and pepper and then scrape the hummus into a small dish.

2 Heat a dry, nonstick frying pan and toast the sesame seeds over a medium-low heat, moving them quickly around the pan until they are golden brown. Stir most of the sesame seeds into the hummus, then sprinkle the rest over the top.

3 Wrap the flatbreads in foil and heat in a preheated oven, 160°C (325°F), Gas Mark 3, for about 10 minutes until warmed through. Drizzle the hummus with olive oil, sprinkle with smoked paprika and serve with the warm flatbreads and crunchy vegetable crudités, if liked.

400 g (13 oz) can chickpeas, rinsed and drained
3 tablespoons lemon juice
1 large garlic clove, crushed
2 tablespoons tahini
1 teaspoon hot smoked paprika, plus extra for sprinkling
½ teaspoon ground cumin
150 ml (¼ pint) extra virgin olive oil, plus extra for drizzling
2 tablespoons sesame seeds
salt and pepper

To serve
4 Lebanese or Turkish flatbreads
crunchy raw vegetable crudités (optional)

Serves **4**
Prep time **15 minutes**
Cooking time **10 minutes**

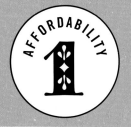

AFFORDABILITY 1

FREEZER AND STORECUPBOARD MEALS

When you're short of time and money, it's time to turn to the freezer and storecupboard for some inspiration. You'll be amazed at the amount of food that gets pushed to the back of freezer drawers or cupboards as new arrivals take pride of place. If you think creatively, there's generally a meal to be made from the cans, packets and cartons that you pull out from the murky depths.

CHILLI CON CARNE

- MINCED BEEF OR LAMB
- ONION AND GARLIC (IF YOU HAVE THEM)
- CHILLI POWDER
- CAN OF KIDNEY BEANS
- CAN OF CHOPPED TOMATOES

Brown the minced meat in a large pan, adding chopped onion and garlic (if you have them). A dash of Worcestershire sauce, barbecue sauce or a stock cube will also give a flavour boost. Add the chilli powder, rinsed and drained kidney beans and the tomatoes and bubble until the meat is cooked through and the sauce reduced. Serve with Boiled Rice (see page 247).

COUSCOUS SALAD

- COUSCOUS
- CAN OF CHICKPEAS
- PAPRIKA
- SUN-DRIED TOMATOES
  (IF YOU HAVE THEM)

Soak the couscous, according to the packet instructions. Add the rinsed and drained chickpeas, a dash of paprika and some chopped sun-dried tomatoes.

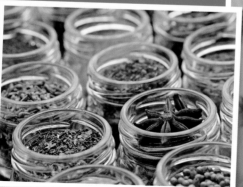

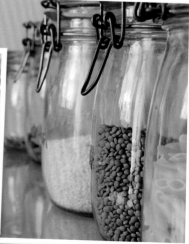

CHICKPEA AND SPINACH CURRY

- SELECTION OF SPICES, SUCH AS CHILLI POWDER, GARAM MASALA, MUSTARD SEEDS, GROUND TURMERIC, GROUND CORIANDER
- ONION
- CAN OF CHICKPEAS
- CAN OF CHOPPED TOMATOES
- HANDFUL OF FROZEN SPINACH

Fry the spices in a little oil, add a chopped onion, then add the rinsed and drained chickpeas and the tomatoes. Cook until the sauce thickens, then add the spinach and heat through. Serve with Boiled Rice (see page 247) or warm naan bread.

TARKA DHAL

- RED LENTILS OR YELLOW SPLIT PEAS, RINSED AND DRAINED
- ONION
- GARLIC
- CHILLI POWDER
- CUMIN SEEDS AND GROUND TURMERIC (IF YOU HAVE THEM)

Cook the lentils according to the packet instructions. Meanwhile, fry a chopped onion, some garlic and the spices in a little oil. Add the spice mix to the lentils and stir to combine.

PILAF

- ONION
- BASMATI RICE
- VEGETABLE OR CHICKEN STOCK CUBE
- FROZEN PEAS

Melt a little butter or oil in a large pan and fry the chopped onion. Add the rice and coat in the oil, then just cover with boiling water and stir in the stock cube. Cover and simmer over a low heat for about 10 minutes or until the rice is cooked. Stir in a handful of frozen peas just before the end of the cooking time. Fluff through the rice with a fork.

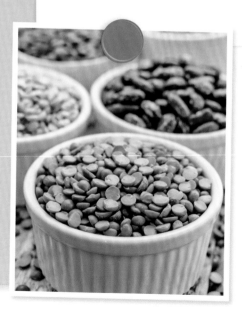

GUACAMOLE

 Vegan

1 Put the avocados and lime juice in a bowl and mash together to prevent discoloration, then stir in the remaining ingredients.

2 Serve immediately with oatcakes or vegetable crudités.

2 ripe avocados, peeled, stoned and chopped
juice of 1 lime
6 cherry tomatoes, diced
1 tablespoon chopped fresh coriander
1–2 garlic cloves, crushed
oatcakes or vegetable crudités, to serve

Serves **4**
Prep time **10 minutes**

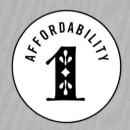

HEALTHY TIP

DOWNLOAD A PEDOMETER There are plenty of free pedometer apps available and this is a great way to check your daily activity. Aim for 10,000 steps a day to help maintain a healthy lifestyle.

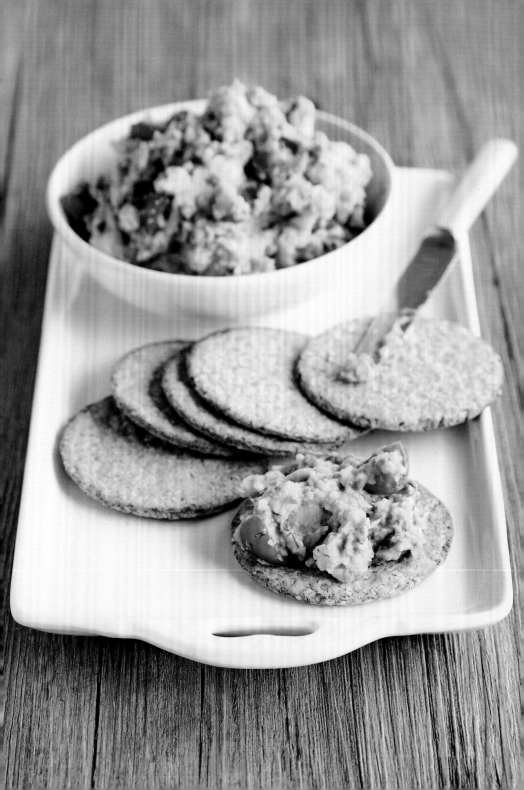

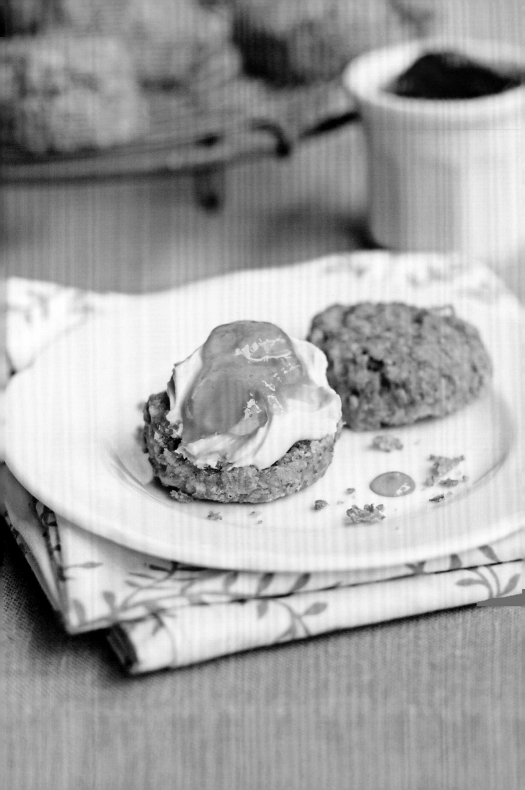

SWEET CARROT & ROSEMARY
SCONES (V)

1   Grease a baking sheet and set aside.

2   Sift the flour, baking powder and cream of tartar into a bowl or food processor, tipping in the grains left in the sieve. Stir in the rosemary and sugar. Add the butter and rub in using your fingertips or process until the mixture resembles breadcrumbs. Stir in the grated carrots and milk and mix or process briefly to make a soft dough, adding a dash more milk if the dough feels dry.

3   Knead the dough on a lightly floured surface until smooth, then roll out to 1.5 cm (¾ inch) thick. Cut out 12 rounds using a 3 cm (1¼ inch) plain biscuit cutter or a glass, re-rolling the trimmings to make more. Place slightly apart on the prepared baking sheet and brush with milk.

4   Bake in a preheated oven, 220°C (425°F), Gas Mark 7, for 8-10 minutes until risen and pale golden. Transfer to a wire rack to cool. Split the scones and serve spread with mascarpone and fruit jelly.

VARIATION
For wholemeal apple and sultana scones, mix 125 g (4 oz) wholemeal plain flour, 100 g (3½ oz) white self-raising flour, 1 teaspoon ground mixed spice and 2 teaspoons baking powder in a bowl or food processor. Add 40 g (1½ oz) slightly salted butter, chilled and diced, and rub in using your fingertips or process until the mixture resembles breadcrumbs. Stir in 50 g (2 oz) chopped sultanas and 1 peeled, cored and grated dessert apple or process briefly. Add 125 ml (4 fl oz) milk and mix or process briefly to make a soft dough, adding a little more milk if the dough feels dry. Roll out, shape and bake as above.

50 g (2 oz) slightly salted butter, chilled and diced, plus extra for greasing
225 g (7½ oz) stoneground spelt flour, plus extra for dusting
2 teaspoons baking powder
½ teaspoon cream of tartar
2 teaspoons finely chopped rosemary
2 tablespoons caster sugar
125 g (4 oz) small carrots, finely grated
100 ml (3½ fl oz) milk, plus extra to glaze

To serve
mascarpone cheese
fruit jelly, such as crab apple, apple or orange

Makes **12**
Prep time **15 minutes, plus cooling**
Cooking time **8-10 minutes**

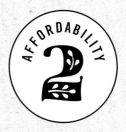

SPICY COURGETTE FRITTERS

1 Grate the courgettes into a colander. Sprinkle lightly with salt and leave for at least 1 hour to drain. Squeeze out the remaining liquid.

2 Place the remaining ingredients, except the eggs and oil, in a mixing bowl and add the grated courgettes. Season lightly with salt and pepper, bearing in mind you have already salted the courgettes, and mix well. Add the eggs and mix again to combine.

3 Heat half of the oil in a large frying pan over a medium-high heat. Place dessertspoonfuls of the mixture (in batches), well spaced, in the pan and press down with the back of the spoon. Cook for 1-2 minutes on each side, until golden and cooked through. Remove from the pan and keep warm. Repeat to cook the rest of the fritters in the same way, adding the remaining oil to the pan when necessary. Serve warm.

ACCOMPANIMENT TIP

For a cucumber, mango and fromage frais relish, to serve as an accompaniment, peel, deseed and coarsely grate 1 cucumber into a fine mesh sieve. Squeeze out any excess liquid using the back of a spoon. Place the grated cucumber in a bowl with 2 tablespoons hot mango chutney and 200 g (7 oz) fat-free fromage frais. Stir in a small handful of finely chopped fresh coriander leaves, season with salt and pepper and chill in the refrigerator until required.

3 courgettes
2 large spring onions, grated or very finely chopped
1 garlic clove, finely chopped
finely grated rind of 1 lemon
4 tablespoons gram flour
2 teaspoons medium curry powder
1 red chilli, deseeded and finely chopped
2 tablespoons finely chopped mint leaves
2 tablespoons finely chopped fresh coriander leaves
2 eggs, lightly beaten
2 tablespoons light olive oil
salt and pepper
cucumber and mango relish, to serve (see Tip)

Serves **4**
Prep time **15 minutes, plus draining**
Cooking time **10-15 minutes**

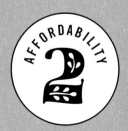

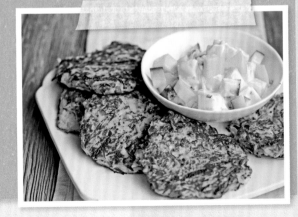

Salmon & Rice BHAJIS

1 Place the salmon, onion, spices, coriander and rice in a large bowl and mix well. Stir in the egg and season well with salt and pepper. Mix in enough of the flour to form a stiff mixture. Using wet hands, shape into 20 small balls.

2 Heat the oil in a large frying pan, add the bhajis and fry for 3-4 minutes, turning once, until golden.

3 Meanwhile, mix together the yogurt, cucumber and mint in a bowl. Serve with the hot bhajis.

2 x 170 g (6 oz) cans salmon, drained and flaked
1 small onion, sliced
½ teaspoon ground cumin
¼ teaspoon dried chilli flakes
2 tablespoons chopped fresh coriander
75 g (3 oz) cooked cold white rice (see page 247)
1 egg, beaten
1-2 tablespoons plain flour
2 tablespoons rapeseed oil
150 ml (¼ pint) natural yogurt
½ cucumber, grated
1 tablespoon chopped mint
salt and pepper

Serves **4**
Prep time **20 minutes**
Cooking time **5 minutes**

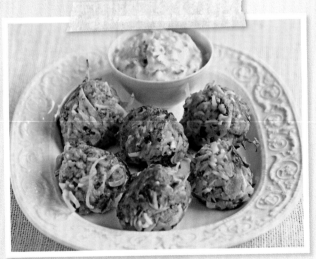

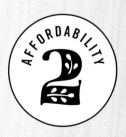

AFFORDABILITY
2

LIGHT **EGG-FRIED** RICE

1 Beat the eggs with the ginger and half of the soy sauce in a bowl until combined.

2 Heat the groundnut oil in a nonstick wok or large frying pan over a high heat until the oil starts to shimmer. Pour in the egg mixture and cook, stirring constantly, for 30 seconds or until softly scrambled.

3 Add the cooked rice, spring onions, sesame oil and remaining soy sauce to the pan and toss together for about 1–2 minutes until the rice is piping hot. Serve immediately.

VARIATION
For fried rice with Chinese leaves and chilli, follow the recipe above, adding 1 deseeded and sliced red chilli and 125 g (4 oz) shredded Chinese leaves once the rice is piping hot, tossing together for a further 30 seconds.

4 eggs
2 teaspoons peeled and finely chopped fresh root ginger
1 ½ tablespoons light soy sauce
2 tablespoons groundnut oil
300 g (10 oz) freshly cooked jasmine rice or long-grain rice (see page 247), cooled
2 spring onions, thinly sliced
¼ teaspoon sesame oil

Serves **4**
Prep time **5 minutes**
Cooking time **5 minutes**

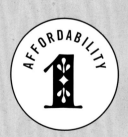

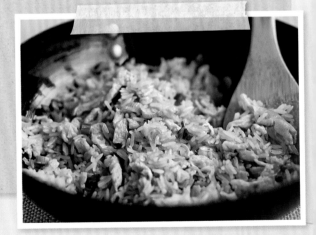

Chilli Kale

1 Heat the oil in a wok or large frying pan over a medium heat. Add the garlic and onion and stir-fry for 5-10 minutes or until the onion is translucent.

2 Add the curly kale and stir-fry for another 5 minutes. Stir in the lime juice and chilli, season with salt and pepper to taste and then serve immediately.

VARIATION
For chilli cabbage, replace the curly kale with 500 g (1 lb) cabbage. Discard the stalks and tough outer leaves, then chop the leaves before frying with the softened garlic and onion, then finishing as above. This recipe also works well with spring greens.

1 tablespoon olive oil
1 garlic clove, crushed
1 large onion, chopped
500 g (1 lb) curly kale, stalks removed and leaves chopped
2 teaspoons lime juice
1 red chilli, deseeded and chopped
salt and pepper

Serves **4**
Prep time **10 minutes**
Cooking time **15 minutes**

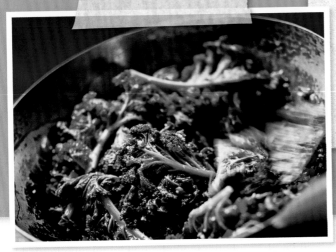

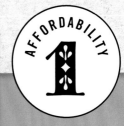

QUICK SPINACH
WITH PINE NUTS

IF YOU HAVE TO WASH THE SPINACH, DO MAKE SURE THAT IT IS DRY BEFORE YOU START TO COOK. PLACE IT IN A SALAD SPINNER OR TEA TOWEL, AND SPIN IT AROUND TO DISPERSE ANY EXCESS WATER.

1 Heat the oil in a large saucepan, add the onion and garlic and sauté for 5 minutes.

2 Put the pine nuts into a small, heavy-based frying pan and dry-fry until browned, stirring constantly as they turn brown very quickly. Remove from the heat.

3 Add the tomatoes, spinach, butter and nutmeg to the onion and garlic and season with salt and pepper. Turn up the heat to high and mix well. Cook for 3 minutes until the spinach has just started to wilt, stirring frequently.

4 Remove from the heat, stir in the pine nuts and serve immediately.

1 tablespoon olive oil
1 red onion, sliced
1 garlic clove, crushed
75 g (3 oz) pine nuts
4 tomatoes, skinned, cored and
   roughly chopped
1 kg (2 lb) spinach, washed and
   trimmed
50 g (2 oz) butter
pinch of freshly grated nutmeg
salt and pepper

Serves **4**
Prep time **10 minutes**
Cooking time **10 minutes**

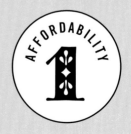

POTATO WEDGES
WITH YOGURT & PARSLEY DIP

1 Cut the potato into 8 wedges and cook them in a saucepan of lightly salted boiling water for 5 minutes. Drain the wedges thoroughly, then put them into a bowl with the red pepper slices and toss with the oil. Sprinkle with paprika and salt to taste.

2 Arrange the potato wedges and pepper slices on a baking tray and cook under a preheated hot grill for 6-8 minutes, turning occasionally, until cooked.

3 Meanwhile, for the yogurt and parsley dip, put the yogurt, parsley, spring onions and garlic, if using, into a bowl. Season to taste with salt and pepper and mix thoroughly.

4 Serve the potato wedges and pepper slices hot with the yogurt dip.

1 potato, about 175 g (6 oz)
1 red pepper, cored, deseeded and sliced
1 teaspoon olive oil
paprika, to taste
salt and pepper

Yogurt and parsley dip
3 tablespoons natural yogurt
1 tablespoon chopped parsley
2 spring onions, chopped
1 garlic clove, crushed (optional)

Serves **1**
Prep time **10 minutes**
Cooking time **15 minutes**

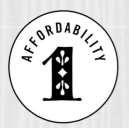

HEALTHY TIP

READ THE LABEL The term *low-fat* can be misleading and you shouldn't automatically assume that these are healthier options. Always read the ingredients list to check what the fat has been replaced with – often the sugar content will be bumped up to compensate.

Healthy MASHED POTATOES (V)

1 Cut the potatoes into chunks and cook in a large saucepan of lightly salted, boiling water for 15-20 minutes until tender. Drain, reserving 2 tablespoons of the cooking water and return the potatoes to the saucepan with the water.

2 Mash well until smooth. Stir in the crème fraîche and plenty of pepper, then serve.

VARIATIONS
Mix and match any of the following ingredients, adding when mashing: finely grated rind of 1 lemon; a handful of finely chopped herbs such as dill, parsley, chervil, tarragon or chives; a couple of tablespoons of chopped (drained) capers or a small garlic clove, finely crushed. You can also use 3-4 tablespoons olive oil or milk instead of the crème fraîche, or swap half of the potatoes for the same weight of parsnips, celeriac or carrots, cooking them in the same pan as the potatoes.

500 g (1 lb) floury potatoes
50 ml (2 fl oz) half-fat crème fraîche
salt and pepper

Serves **2**
Prep time **10 minutes**
Cooking time **15-20 minutes**

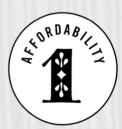

AFFORDABILITY 1

COURGETTE
& RICOTTA BAKES

1 Grease 8 holes of a muffin tin.

2 Use a vegetable peeler to make 16 long ribbons of courgette and set aside. Coarsely grate the remaining courgettes and squeeze to remove any excess moisture. Mix the grated courgettes with all the remaining ingredients in a bowl and season well with salt and pepper.

3 Arrange 2 courgette ribbons in a cross shape in each hole of the prepared muffin tin. Spoon in the filling and then fold over the overhanging courgette ends. Bake in a preheated oven, 190°C (375°F), Gas Mark 5, for 15-20 minutes or until golden and cooked through. Turn out on to serving plates and serve immediately.

VARIATION

For mushrooms stuffed with courgettes and ricotta, brush a little olive oil over 4 large field mushrooms, trimmed, and place on a baking tray, stalk side up. Grate 1 courgette and squeeze to remove any excess moisture, then mix with 200 g (7 oz) ricotta cheese, 4 drained and chopped sun-dried tomatoes in oil and 25 g (1 oz) chopped pitted black olives. Season with salt and pepper, spoon on to the mushrooms, then sprinkle with 25 g (1 oz) grated Parmesan-style cheese. Bake in a preheated oven, 200°C (400°F), Gas Mark 6, for 15 minutes until golden and cooked through. Serve with ciabatta rolls.

butter, for greasing
2 courgettes
100 g (3½ oz) fresh white or
    wholemeal breadcrumbs
250 g (8 oz) ricotta cheese
75 g (3 oz) Parmesan-style cheese,
    grated
2 eggs, beaten
1 garlic clove, crushed
handful of chopped basil
salt and pepper

Serves **4**
Prep time **15 minutes**
Cooking time **15-20 minutes**

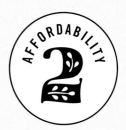

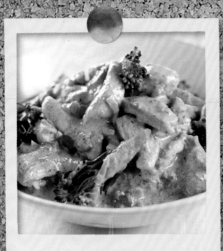

FAST CHICKEN CURRY

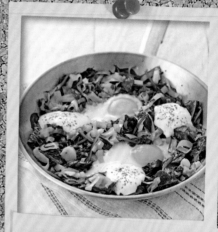

PAN-COOKED EGGS
WITH SPINACH & LEEKS

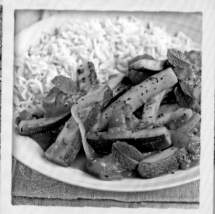

LEBANESE TOMATO
& COURGETTE CURRY

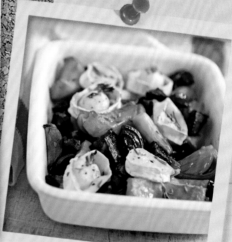

PUMPKIN & GOATS' CHEESE BAKE

Make it Light

ONE-POT CHICKEN

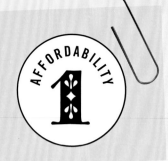

1 Place the potatoes in a saucepan of boiling water and cook for 12-15 minutes until tender. Drain, then cut into bite-sized pieces.

2 Make a slit lengthways down the side of each chicken breast to form a pocket, ensuring that you do not cut all the way through. Mix together the herbs, garlic and crème fraîche, season well with pepper, then spoon a little of the mixture into each chicken pocket.

3 Put the leeks, chicory and potatoes in an ovenproof dish. Pour over the stock, then lay the chicken breasts on top. Spoon over the remaining crème fraîche mixture, then bake in a preheated oven, 200°C (400°F), Gas Mark 6, for 25-30 minutes or until the chicken is cooked through. Serve immediately.

VARIATION

For baked chicken with fennel and potatoes, cut the cooked potatoes in half and place them in a large ovenproof dish with 1 large fennel bulb, cut into quarters. Omit the leeks and chicory. Pour over the stock and bake in a preheated oven at 200°C (400°F), Gas Mark 6, for 20 minutes. Remove from the oven and lay the un-filled chicken breasts over the vegetables. Combine 1 tablespoon chopped parsley with 1 tablespoon Dijon mustard and the half-fat crème fraîche, omitting the garlic, and spoon the mixture over the chicken. Bake for a further 25-30 minutes until the chicken is cooked through. Calories per serving 279

500 g (1 lb) new potatoes
4 chicken breasts, about 125 g (4 oz) each
6 tablespoons chopped mixed herbs, such as parsley, chives, chervil and mint
1 garlic clove, crushed
6 tablespoons half-fat crème fraîche
8 baby leeks, trimmed and cleaned
2 chicory heads, halved lengthways
150 ml (¼ pint) Chicken Stock (see page 244)
pepper

Calories per serving **275**
Serves **4**
Prep time **10 minutes**
Cooking time **40-45 minutes**

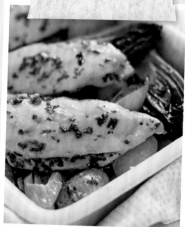

SPICED ROAST CHICKEN
with lime

1 Cut a few slashes across each chicken thigh. Mix together the harissa and honey and rub all over the chicken thighs. Place in a roasting tin large enough to spread everything out in a single layer, with the lime wedges, red pepper, courgettes, onion and potatoes.

2 Drizzle over the oil, season with salt and pepper, then roast in a preheated oven, 220°C (425°F), Gas Mark 7, for 25 minutes, turning occasionally, or until the chicken is cooked and the vegetables are tender. Serve with the juice of the lime wedges squeezed over the chicken.

VARIATION
For pan-fried spicy chicken, cut 8 small boneless, skinless chicken thighs into strips and coat in a mixture of 1 tablespoon harissa and 1 tablespoon clear honey. Heat 1 tablespoon sunflower oil in a large frying pan, add the chicken and fry over a medium heat for 5 minutes. Add 1 cored, deseeded and chopped red pepper, 2 chopped courgettes, 1 onion, cut into thin wedges, and 2 limes, cut into wedges. Cook for 10 minutes, stirring occasionally, or until the chicken is cooked through and the vegetables are tender. Serve with new potatoes. Calories per serving 316

8 small (bone-in) chicken thighs, skinned
1 tablespoon harissa
4 tablespoons clear honey
2 limes, cut into wedges
1 red pepper, cored, deseeded and cut into large chunks
2 courgettes, cut into chunks
1 onion, cut into wedges
300 g (10 oz) new potatoes, halved if large
1 tablespoon olive oil
salt and pepper

Calories per serving **362**
Serves **4**
Prep time **15 minutes**
Cooking time **25 minutes**

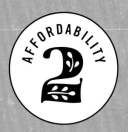

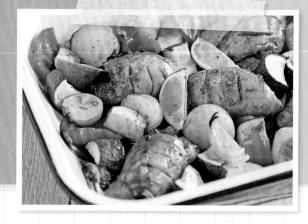

Fast Chicken CURRY

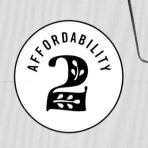

1   Heat the oil in a nonstick saucepan over a medium heat. Add the onion and cook for 3 minutes until softened and translucent. Add the curry paste and cook, stirring, for 1 minute until fragrant.

2   Add the chicken, tomatoes, broccoli and coconut milk to the pan. Bring to the boil, then reduce the heat, cover and simmer gently over a low heat, stirring occasionally, for 15–20 minutes until the chicken is cooked through.

3   Season well with salt and pepper and serve immediately.

VARIATION

For chicken patties with curry sauce, follow the first stage of the recipe above, then add the tomatoes, 200 g (7 oz) baby spinach leaves and the reduced-fat coconut milk (omitting the chicken and broccoli), and cook as directed. Meanwhile, finely chop 450 g (14½ oz) cooked boneless, skinless chicken breasts. Transfer to a bowl and add 4 finely chopped spring onions, 2 tablespoons chopped fresh coriander, 50 g (2 oz) fresh white or wholemeal breadcrumbs, a squeeze of lemon juice and 1 beaten egg. Season with salt and pepper. Mix well, then form into 16 patties. Roll in 25 g (1 oz) fresh white or wholemeal breadcrumbs to coat. Brush a large frying pan with a little vegetable oil and heat over a medium heat. Add the patties, cooking in batches, and pan-fry on each side until golden brown and cooked through. Serve hot with the curry sauce. Calories per serving 490

3 tablespoons olive oil
1 onion, finely chopped
4 tablespoons medium curry paste
8 boneless, skinless chicken thighs, cut into thin strips
400 g (13 oz) can chopped tomatoes
250 g (8 oz) broccoli, broken into small florets, stalks peeled and sliced
100 ml (3½ fl oz) reduced-fat coconut milk
salt and pepper

Calories per serving **413**
Serves **4**
Prep time **10 minutes**
Cooking time **20-25 minutes**

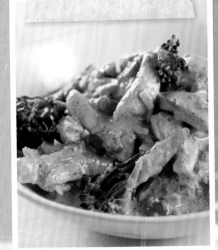

DEVILLED CHICKEN

1 Remove the skin from the chicken thighs, open them out and trim away any fat. Mix together the mustard, Tabasco, garlic and soy sauce in a shallow dish.

2 Heat a large griddle pan or nonstick frying pan until hot.

3 Dip the trimmed chicken thighs in the devil sauce and coat each piece well. Place the chicken pieces flat on the hot pan and cook for 8–10 minutes on each side. Serve hot or cold with a mixed leaf salad.

VARIATION
For jerk chicken, mix 3 tablespoons jerk marinade (a ready-made paste) with the finely grated rind and juice of ½ orange and 2 finely chopped garlic cloves. Dip the chicken in this mixture then cook as above. Serve with Boiled Rice (see page 247) or a salad. Calories per serving 203

8 small-medium, boneless chicken thighs
2 tablespoons Dijon mustard
6 drops of Tabasco sauce
2 garlic cloves, crushed
1 tablespoon soy sauce
mixed leaf salad, to serve

Calories per serving **207**
Serves **4**
Prep time **10 minutes**
Cooking time **20 minutes**

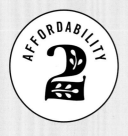

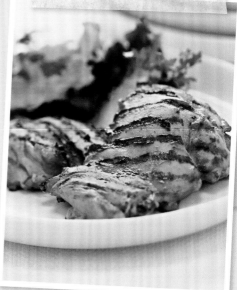

LOW-FAT **LEMON CHICKEN**

1   Mix together the egg, garlic and lemon rind in a shallow glass or ceramic dish. Add the chicken and toss to coat evenly, then cover and leave to marinate at room temperature for 10–15 minutes.

2   Discard the lemon rind, then add the cornflour to the marinated chicken. Mix well to distribute the cornflour evenly between the chicken slices.

3   Heat the oil in a nonstick wok or large frying pan over a high heat until the oil starts to shimmer. Add the chicken slices, making sure you leave a little space between them, and fry for 2 minutes on each side.

4   Reduce the heat to medium and stir-fry for a further 1 minute or until the chicken is browned and cooked through. Increase the heat and pour in the lemon juice. Stir in the spring onion, then garnish with lemon slices and serve immediately with boiled rice.

VARIATION
For warm lemon chicken and herb salad, cook the chicken as above, then toss in a bowl with ½ cucumber, sliced, a handful of fresh coriander leaves, 6 torn basil leaves and 50 g (2 oz) rocket leaves. Dress the salad lightly with ½ teaspoon sesame oil and 1 teaspoon rapeseed or olive oil. Calories per serving 263

1 egg, lightly beaten
2 garlic cloves, sliced
2 small pieces of lemon rind, plus the juice of 1 lemon
500 g (1 lb) skinless chicken breast fillets, cut into 5 mm (¼ inch) slices
2 tablespoons cornflour
1 tablespoon rapeseed or olive oil
1 spring onion, diagonally sliced into 1.5 cm (¾ inch) lengths
lemon slices, to garnish
Boiled Rice (see page 247), to serve

Calories per serving **417**
Serves **4**
Prep time **15 minutes, plus marinating**
Cooking time **8 minutes**

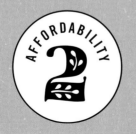

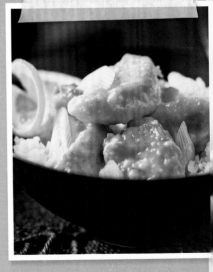

Chicken
WITH ORANGE & MINT

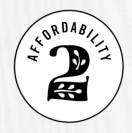

1 Season the chicken breasts with salt and pepper. Heat the oil in a large nonstick frying pan, add the chicken breasts and cook over a medium heat, turning once, for 4–5 minutes or until golden all over.

2 Pour in the orange juice, add the orange slices, then bring to a gentle simmer. Cover tightly, reduce the heat to low and cook gently for 8–10 minutes or until the chicken is cooked through. Add the mint and butter and stir to mix well. Cook over a high heat, stirring, for 2 minutes. Serve with steamed couscous, if liked.

VARIATION

For chicken with rosemary and lemon, bruise 4 sprigs of rosemary using a pestle and mortar, then chop finely. Put the grated rind and juice of 2 lemons, 3 crushed garlic cloves, 4 tablespoons olive oil and the rosemary in a non-metallic dish. Add the chicken breasts and mix to coat thoroughly. Cover and leave to marinate in the refrigerator for at least 30 mins or overnight. Cook the chicken breasts in a preheated hot ridged griddle pan for 5 minutes on each side or until cooked through. Calories per serving 370

4 boneless, skinless chicken breasts, about 200 g (7 oz) each
3 tablespoons olive oil
150 ml (¼ pint) freshly squeezed orange juice
1 small orange, sliced
2 tablespoons chopped mint
1 tablespoon butter
salt and pepper
steamed couscous (approximately 2 tablespoons per serving), to serve (optional)

Calories per serving **355 (excluding couscous)**
Serves **4**
Prep time **5 minutes**
Cooking time **15–20 minutes**

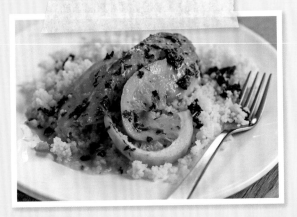

CALVES' LIVER
with garlic mash

1 Cook the potatoes and garlic in a saucepan of lightly salted boiling water for 10-12 minutes until tender, then drain. Return the potatoes and garlic to the pan and mash with the crème fraîche and sage. Season well with pepper.

2 Meanwhile, press the pieces of liver into the seasoned flour to coat them all over. Heat the oil in a non-stick frying pan until hot, add the liver slices and fry for 1-2 minutes on each side or until cooked to your liking. Serve with the garlic mash and gravy.

350 g (11 ½ oz) potatoes, cubed
1 garlic clove, peeled
3 tablespoons half-fat crème fraîche
1½ teaspoons chopped sage
2 slices of calves liver, about 150 g (5 oz) each
1 tablespoon plain flour, seasoned with salt and pepper
1½ teaspoons olive oil
salt and pepper
Gravy (see page 245), to serve

Calories per serving **393**
Serves **2**
Prep time **10 minutes**
Cooking time **12-16 minutes**

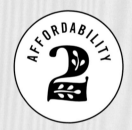

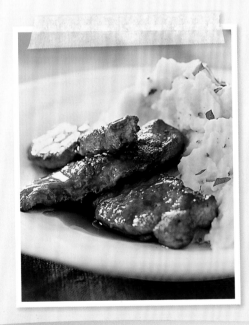

BEEF
IN BLACK BEAN SAUCE

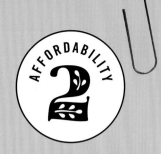

AFFORDABILITY 2

1 Heat 1 tablespoon of the oil in a nonstick wok over a high heat until the oil starts to shimmer. Add half of the beef, season with salt and stir-fry for 2 minutes. When it begins to colour, lift the beef on to a plate using a slotted spoon. Heat another 1 tablespoon of the oil and stir-fry the rest of the beef in the same way.

2 Return the wok to the heat and wipe it clean with kitchen paper. Heat the remaining oil and tip in the red pepper, sweetcorn, chilli and shallots. Stir-fry for 2 minutes before adding the black bean sauce, water and cornflour paste.

3 Bring to the boil, stirring, then return the beef to the wok and stir-fry until the sauce thickens and coats the ingredients in a velvety glaze. Serve with boiled rice, if liked.

VARIATION

For king prawns with spring onions and black bean sauce, replace the beef with 250 g (8 oz) raw peeled king prawns. Replace the sweetcorn, green chilli and shallots with 75 g (3 oz) bean sprouts, 1 red chilli deseeded and cut into strips, and 3 spring onions cut into 1 cm (½ inch) pieces, and cook as above. Calories per serving 171 (excluding rice)

3 tablespoons groundnut oil
500 g (1 lb) lean beef, cut into thin slices
1 red pepper, cored, deseeded and cut into strips
6 baby sweetcorn, cut in half lengthways
1 green chilli, deseeded and cut into strips
3 shallots, cut into thin wedges
2 tablespoons black bean sauce
4 tablespoons water
1 teaspoon cornflour mixed to a paste with 1 tablespoon water
salt
Boiled Rice (see page 247), to serve (optional)

Calories per serving **294 (excluding rice)**
Serves **4**
Prep time **15 minutes**
Cooking time **10 minutes**

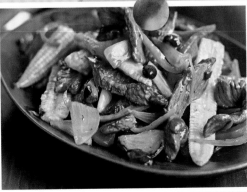

LEAN LASAGNE

1. To make the meat sauce, put the aubergines, onions, garlic, stock and wine in a large saucepan. Cover, bring to the boil, then simmer briskly for 5 minutes. Remove the lid and cook for a further 5 minutes or until the aubergines are tender and the liquid is absorbed, adding a little more stock if necessary. Remove from the heat and leave to cool slightly, then purée in a blender or food processor.

2. Meanwhile, brown the minced beef in a nonstick frying pan. Skim off any fat. Add the aubergine mixture and the tomatoes and season with pepper. Simmer briskly, uncovered, stirring occasionally, for about 10 minutes until thickened.

3. Make the cheese sauce. Beat the egg whites with the ricotta in a bowl, then beat in the milk and 4 tablespoons of the Parmesan. Season with pepper.

4. Alternate layers of the meat sauce, lasagne and cheese sauce in a 1.5 litre (2 ¾ pint) ovenproof dish, starting with meat sauce and finishing with cheese sauce. Sprinkle the top with the remaining Parmesan. Bake in a preheated oven, 180°C (350°F), Gas Mark 4, for 30–40 minutes until browned. Serve hot.

200 g (7 oz) pre-cooked lasagne sheets

Meat sauce
2 aubergines, peeled and diced
2 red onions, chopped
2 garlic cloves, crushed
300 ml (½ pint) Vegetable Stock (see page 244)
4 tablespoons red wine
500 g (1 lb) extra-lean minced beef
2 x 400 g (13 oz) cans chopped tomatoes
pepper

Cheese sauce
3 egg whites
250 g (8 oz) ricotta cheese
175 ml (6 fl oz) milk
6 tablespoons grated Parmesan cheese

Calories per serving **340**
Serves **8**
Prep time **30 minutes**
Cooking time **50–60 minutes**

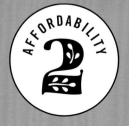

AFFORDABILITY 2

GRILLED SARDINES
WITH TABBOULEH

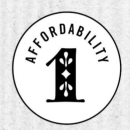

1 Cook the bulgar wheat in a small saucepan of boiling water for 5 minutes, then drain and refresh under cold running water. Drain again and put into a bowl.

2 Meanwhile, dry-fry the onion in a small, nonstick frying pan for 5 minutes. Put the tomatoes in a heatproof bowl and pour over enough boiling water to cover, then leave for about 1 minute. Drain, skin the tomatoes, then deseed and finely chop the flesh.

3 Add the onion, tomatoes, lemon juice and lemon rind to the bulgar wheat. Reserve 4 mint leaves, then chop the rest. Stir the chopped mint into the bulgar wheat mixture and season with salt and pepper.

4 Open out each sardine and lay a mint leaf along the centre. Spoon over a little of the tabbouleh and carefully fold each fillet back over. Cook the sardines under a preheated hot grill for 5 minutes, then carefully turn them over and cook for a further 5 minutes or until cooked through. Serve with the remaining tabbouleh (hot or cold), lemon wedges and a few salad or herb leaves.

125 g (4 oz) bulgar wheat
1 onion, finely chopped
2 ripe tomatoes
1 tablespoon lemon juice
1 teaspoon finely grated lemon rind
small handful of mint leaves
4 small sardines, gutted and boned
salt and pepper

To serve
lemon wedges
salad or herb leaves

Calories per serving **209**
Serves **4**
Prep time **15 minutes**
Cooking time **15 minutes**

STEAMED GINGER FISH

1 Pat the fish dry with kitchen paper and season well with salt and white pepper. Place in a single layer on a heatproof plate that will fit inside a bamboo steamer and scatter evenly with the ginger, chilli and orange and lemon rinds.

2 Place the plate in the bamboo steamer, cover and steam over a wok or large saucepan of boiling water for about 6-8 minutes until the fish is just cooked through – the flesh should be opaque in the centre and slightly flaking but still moist.

3 Remove the plate from the steamer and drain off any liquid that may have accumulated around the fish. Scatter the spring onions over the fish, then drizzle with the soy sauce and sprinkle over the chopped coriander. Serve with stir-fry vegetable rice (see Tip) or boiled rice and steamed Asian greens.

ACCOMPANIMENT TIP
For stir-fry vegetable rice, to serve as an accompaniment, spray a large nonstick wok or frying pan with low-calorie cooking spray and place over a high heat until almost smoking. Add 500 g (1 lb) cooled freshly cooked jasmine rice and stir-fry for 3 minutes. Add a 400 g (13 oz) packet mixed prepared stir-fry vegetables and stir-fry for 5 minutes. Season well with salt and pepper, then stir in 2 tablespoons light soy sauce and 4 thinly sliced spring onions and stir-fry for a further 2 minutes. Serve immediately. Calories per serving 256

4 thick-cut halibut or cod fillets, about 200 g (7 oz) each
thumb-sized piece of fresh root ginger, peeled and finely shredded
1 red chilli, deseeded and finely shredded
1 tablespoon finely grated orange rind
1 tablespoon finely grated lemon rind
2 spring onions, finely shredded
2 tablespoons light soy sauce
1 tablespoon finely chopped fresh coriander leaves
salt and white pepper
Stir-fry Vegetable Rice (see Tip) or Boiled Rice (see page 247) and steamed Asian greens, to serve

Calories per serving **179 (excluding rice)**
Serves **4**
Prep time **15 minutes**
Cooking time **6-8 minutes**

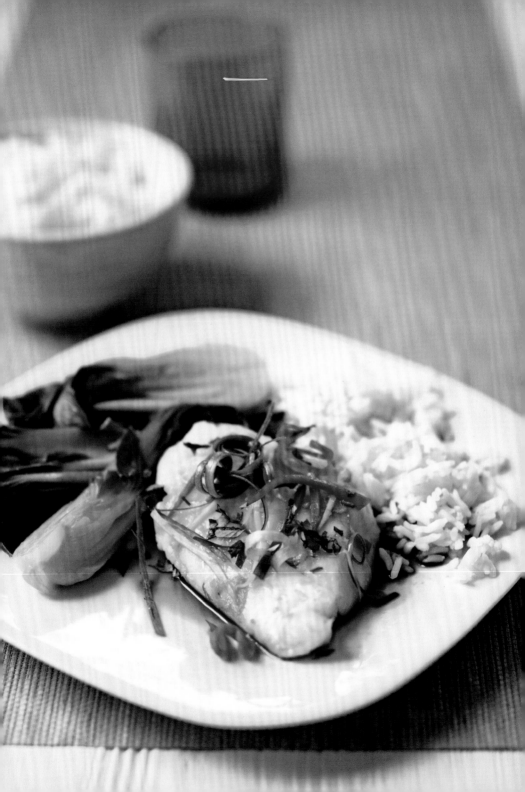

CHILLI & CORIANDER
FISH PARCEL

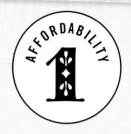
1 Place the fish in a non-metallic dish and sprinkle with the lemon juice. Cover and leave to marinate in the refrigerator for 15-20 minutes.

2 Place the coriander, garlic and chilli in a mini food processor and process until the mixture forms a paste. Add the sugar and yogurt and briefly process to combine.

3 Lay the fish fillet on a sheet of nonstick baking paper or foil and coat on both sides with the paste. Gather up the baking paper or foil loosely around the fish and turn over at the top to seal. Chill in the refrigerator for at least 1 hour.

4 Place the parcel on a baking tray and bake in a preheated oven, 200°C (400°F), Gas Mark 6, for about 15 minutes or until the fish is just cooked through. Serve garnished with extra coriander and chilli.

125 g (4 oz) cod, coley or haddock fillet
2 teaspoons lemon juice
1 tablespoon chopped fresh coriander leaves, plus extra to garnish
1 garlic clove, peeled
1 green chilli, deseeded and chopped, plus extra to garnish
¼ teaspoon sugar
2 teaspoons natural yogurt

Calories per serving **127**
Serves **1**
Prep time **15 minutes, plus marinating and chilling**
Cooking time **15 minutes**

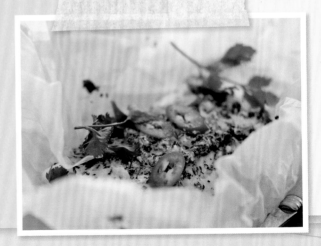

SQUID, PEPPER & RED RICE
PILAF

1 Slice the squid into rings. Toast the almonds in a dry frying pan and slide out on to a plate. Heat the oil in the pan and gently fry the green peppers for 5 minutes to soften. Push the peppers to one side of the pan, add the squid rings and fry for 3 minutes until plumped up. Transfer the squid to a plate and set aside, leaving the peppers in the pan.

2 Add the onion and celery to the pan and fry for a further 5 minutes until all the vegetables start to colour. Add the garlic and fry for 1 minute.

3 Stir in the rice and stock. Cook very gently, stirring frequently, for about 25 minutes or until the rice is tender. Add more hot water if the liquid has evaporated before the rice is tender.

4 Return the squid to the pan with the coriander and heat through gently for 2 minutes or until the squid is hot. Season to taste with salt and pepper and serve.

200 g (7 oz) squid tubes
25 g (1 oz) flaked almonds
1 tablespoon olive oil
2 green peppers, cored, deseeded
  and roughly chopped
1 red onion, thinly sliced
2 celery sticks, chopped
2 garlic cloves, crushed
150 g (5 oz) red rice
600 ml (1 pint) Vegetable or
  Chicken Stock (see pages 244)
2 tablespoons chopped fresh
  coriander
salt and pepper

Calories per serving **364**
Serves **2**
Prep time **15 minutes**
Cooking time **45 minutes**

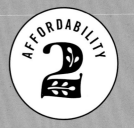

AFFORDABILITY
2

KERALAN-STYLE MUSSELS

1 Scrub the mussels, scraping off any barnacles and pulling away the beards. Discard any damaged shells or open ones that do not close when tapped firmly against the side of the sink.

2 Melt the butter in a large saucepan and gently fry the onion for 2 minutes. Add the garlic, cardamom pods, tamarind paste and curry leaves and fry for 30 seconds. Add the tomatoes and stock and bring to the boil.

3 Tip in the mussels and cover with a lid. Cook for about 5 minutes, shaking the pan frequently until the shells have opened. Using a slotted spoon, drain the mussels to serving dishes (discarding any unopened mussels) and keep warm.

4 Add the coconut to the pan and heat through until almost boiling. Season to taste with salt and pepper, then spoon over the mussels to serve. Serve with warm grainy bread.

1 kg (2 lb) fresh mussels
15 g (½ oz) butter
1 onion, finely chopped
3 garlic cloves, crushed
10 cardamom pods, crushed
1 teaspoon tamarind paste
6 curry leaves
2 tomatoes, skinned, deseeded
 and chopped
100 ml (3½ fl oz) fish stock or
 Vegetable Stock (see page 244)
150 ml (¼ pint) creamed coconut
salt and pepper
warm grainy bread, to serve

Calories per serving **446**
Serves **2**
Prep time **20 minutes**
Cooking time **10 minutes**

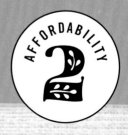

AFFORDABILITY
2

STIR-FRIED TOFU
WITH BASIL & CHILLI

1 Heat half of the oil in a nonstick wok or deep frying pan until smoking, then add the tofu and stir-fry for 2–3 minutes until golden all over. Remove to a plate with a slotted spoon.

2 Add the remaining oil to the pan with the ginger and garlic and stir-fry for 10 seconds, then add the broccoli and sugar snap peas and stir-fry for 1 minute.

3 Return the tofu to the pan and then add the stock, chilli sauce, soy sauces, lime juice and sugar. Stir-fry for 1 minute until the vegetables are cooked but still crisp. Add the basil leaves, stir well, then serve.

VARIATION
For tofu and vegetables in oyster sauce, cook the tofu and vegetables as above. Return the tofu to the pan and add 50 ml (2 fl oz) water, cook for 1 minute, then add 75 ml (3 fl oz) oyster sauce and heat through for a further 1 minute. Omit the basil and garnish with chopped fresh coriander.
Calories per serving 244

2 tablespoons sunflower oil
350 g (11½ oz) firm tofu, drained and cubed
5 cm (2 inch) piece of fresh root ginger, peeled and grated
2 garlic cloves, chopped
250 g (8 oz) broccoli, trimmed
250 g (8 oz) sugar snap peas, trimmed
150 ml (¼ pint) Vegetable Stock (see page 244)
2 tablespoons sweet chilli sauce
1 tablespoon light soy sauce
1 tablespoon dark soy sauce
1 tablespoon lime juice
2 teaspoons soft light brown sugar
handful of Thai basil leaves

Calories per serving **273**
Serves **4**
Prep time **20 minutes**
Cooking time **10 minutes**

AFFORDABILITY 1

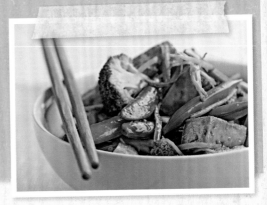

Takeaway Alternatives

There's nothing quite as satisfying as settling down to a night in front of the telly with a takeaway winging its way to your front door. With pretty much every cuisine now just a phone call or mouse click away, you can indulge your cravings for everything from a pizza to a pie without having to lift a finger in the kitchen. However, while you might enjoy tucking into a takeaway, it will have a serious impact on your waistline and wallet.

Part of the appeal of dialling in an order for dinner is that you don't have to cook, but it's worth considering the fact that for the price of your tikka masala and trimmings, you could rustle up an equivalent feast for your whole household. So, here are some quick and easy alternatives to popular takeaway treats.

FISH AND CHIPS

Homemade oven chips are just as tasty as those from your local chippy and if you cut out the batter from the fish by grilling a nice piece of cod or haddock, you've turned a fat-charged Friday supper into something more amenable to a healthy lifestyle. You can even make a pea purée by yes, quite literally, puréeing cooked peas.

THAI CURRY

You'll need an authentic red or green curry paste to make this rival the real thing. Fry chopped onion and strips of boneless, skinless chicken thigh meat until browned, stir in the curry paste, add the required amount of coconut milk and stir until the chicken is cooked through. Serve with sticky or jasmine rice.

EGG-FRIED RICE

Cook the amount of rice you require and drain, then heat a little oil in a large pan. Fry off some chopped onion and add mushrooms, frozen (defrosted) peas, grated ginger and garlic, if you like. Whisk a couple of eggs and pour into the pan, then use the spatula to break them up as they cook. Add the rice to the pan, stir until all the ingredients are combined, then dish up.

KEBABS

This quick, healthy alternative to the high street doner will be a hit with your housemates. Thread diced boneless, skinless chicken breast (or thigh meat) and cored, deseeded chunks of red pepper on to pre-soaked wooden skewers and grill until cooked through. Meanwhile, warm pitta breads or Turkish pides, load up with shredded lettuce and hummus and then pile the chicken and peppers on top.

PIZZA

You can use shop-bought pizza bases or better still make your own dough. Alternatively, flatbreads, wraps and naan bread all make great bases. Spread over a layer of passata (sieved tomatoes), then add grated cheese and other toppings of your choice, such as sliced pepper, red chilli, cooked chicken, mushrooms, lean ham, etc. Cook in a hot oven for about 5–8 minutes... it's literally that simple.

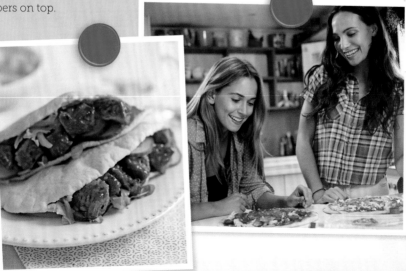

SPINACH & PEA FRITTATA

1 Heat the oil in a heavy-based, nonstick, ovenproof 23 cm (9 inch) frying pan over a low heat. Add the onion and cook, stirring occasionally, for 6-8 minutes until softened, then stir in the spinach and peas and cook for a further 2 minutes or until any moisture released by the spinach has evaporated.

2 Beat the eggs in a bowl and season lightly with salt and pepper. Stir in the cooked vegetables, then pour the mixture back into the frying pan and quickly arrange the vegetables so that they are evenly dispersed. Cook over a low heat for 8-10 minutes or until all but the top of the frittata is set.

3 Transfer the frying pan to a preheated very hot grill and cook about 10 cm (4 inches) from the heat source until the top is set but not coloured. Give the pan a shake to loosen the frittata, then transfer to a plate to cool. Serve slightly warm or at room temperature, accompanied by a green salad, if liked.

VARIATION
For a courgette, pea and cheese frittata, follow the first step as above, but replace the spinach with 1 large courgette, coarsely grated. Add 4 tablespoons grated Parmesan-style cheese and 100 g (3½ oz) cubed mozzarella cheese to the raw egg mixture with the vegetables and cook as above. Calories per serving 312

1 tablespoon olive oil
1 onion, thinly sliced
150 g (5 oz) baby spinach leaves
125 g (4 oz) shelled fresh or frozen peas
6 eggs
salt and pepper
green salad, to serve (optional)

Calories per serving **201 (excluding green salad)**
Serves **4**
Prep time **10 minutes, plus cooling**
Cooking time **25 minutes**

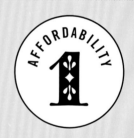

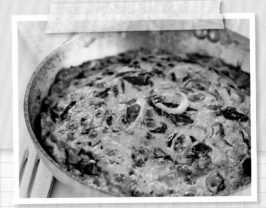

Sweet Potato, Red Onion & Dill
FRITTATA

1. Heat the oil in a nonstick frying pan about 22 cm (8½ inches) in diameter. Add the onions and sweet potatoes and fry very gently for 10-15 minutes until softened and pale golden. Stir the vegetables frequently to prevent them over browning.

2. Whisk the eggs in a bowl to break up. Beat in the dill and a little salt and pepper.

3. Reduce the heat to its lowest setting and pour the eggs evenly over the vegetables in the pan. Cook very gently for a couple of minutes, pushing the cooked egg mixture from the edges of the pan in towards the centre. Once partially cooked, cover the pan with foil or a lid and cook for a further 3-4 minutes or until the eggs are lightly set.

4. Leave to cool slightly, turn out on to a plate and serve warm or leave to cool completely before serving.

3 tablespoons olive oil
2 red onions, thinly sliced
500 g (1 lb) sweet potatoes, scrubbed and cut into 2 cm (¾ inch) chunks
5 eggs
3 tablespoons chopped dill
salt and pepper

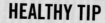

Calories per serving **636**
Serves **2**
Prep time **10 minutes, plus cooling**
Cooking time **20 minutes**

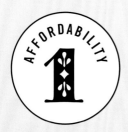

AFFORDABILITY
1

HEALTHY TIP

CUT DOWN ON CAFFEINE There's nothing wrong with the odd cup of coffee to get your through a tedious late-afternoon lecture. But if there's a caffeine hit in your hand every break, it's time to cut down. Try switching every other coffee for a peppermint or green tea.

PAN-COOKED EGGS
WITH SPINACH & LEEKS

1 Melt the butter in a frying pan, add the leek and chilli flakes and cook over a medium-high heat for 4–5 minutes until softened. Add the spinach and season well with salt and pepper, then toss and cook for 2 minutes until wilted.

2 Make 2 wells in the centre of the vegetables and break an egg into each well. Cook over a low heat for 2–3 minutes until the eggs are set. Spoon the yogurt on top and sprinkle with the paprika, then serve

25 g (1 oz) butter
1 leek, trimmed, cleaned and thinly sliced
¼ teaspoon dried chilli flakes
300 g (10 oz) baby spinach leaves
2 eggs
3 tablespoons natural yogurt
pinch of ground paprika
salt and pepper

Calories per serving **265**
Serves **2**
Prep time **10 minutes**
Cooking time **10 minutes**

HEALTHY TIP

ALCOHOL FREE If you want a clear head in the morning, alternate your regular lager with bottles of low alcohol or alcohol-free brands — there are some fairly authentic varieties on the market these days.

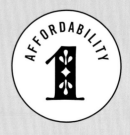

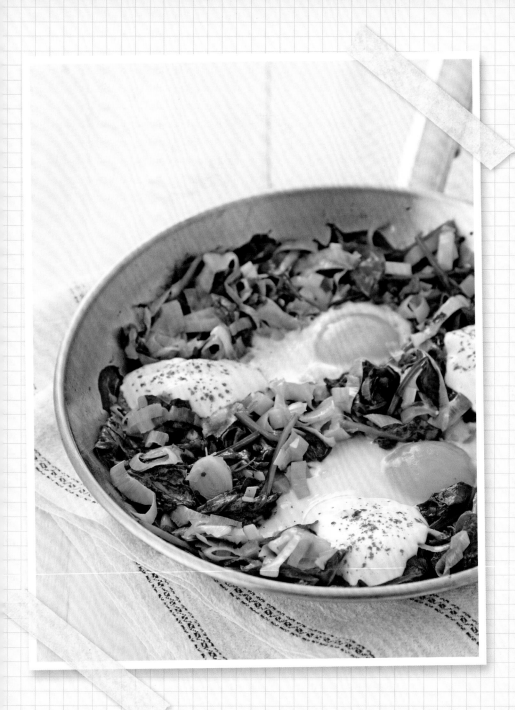

TOMATO & HERB PIZZA PIE

1 Lightly grease a baking sheet and set aside.

2 Make the scone base. Sift the flour into a mixing bowl, tipping in the grain left in the sieve, then rub in the spread until the mixture resembles fine breadcrumbs. Add just enough milk to make a soft dough. Turn out on to a lightly floured surface and knead until smooth. Roll out to a 23-25 cm (9-10 inch) diameter round, then place on the prepared baking sheet.

3 For the topping, heat the oil in a large, nonstick saucepan, add the onion and garlic and fry gently for 5 minutes until softened. Add the green or red pepper, tomatoes, tomato purée and basil or thyme and simmer, uncovered, stirring occasionally, for about 10 minutes until the mixture is thick. Season with pepper.

4 Spread the tomato mixture over the scone base to the edge. Top with the mozzarella cheese. Bake in a preheated oven, 220°C (425°F), Gas Mark 7, for 20-25 minutes until the topping is bubbling. Garnish with basil sprigs and serve.

VARIATION
For the topping, you could instead try: anchovy fillets and black olives; red onion, feta cheese, red pepper and rocket; spinach and ricotta.

50 g (2 oz) unsaturated spread, plus extra for greasing
300 g (10 oz) wholemeal self-raising flour, plus extra for dusting
150 ml (¼ pint) skimmed milk

Topping
1 tablespoon olive oil
2 large onions, chopped
1-2 garlic cloves, crushed
1 green or red pepper, cored, deseeded and sliced
2 x 400 g (13 oz) cans tomatoes
2 tablespoons tomato purée
large handful of basil or thyme, chopped
125 g (4 oz) half-fat mozzarella cheese, sliced
pepper
basil sprigs, to garnish

Calories per serving **340**
Serves **6**
Prep time **15 minutes**
Cooking time **35-40 minutes**

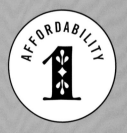

HEALTHY TIP
Home-made pizzas can be very healthy, with a starchy base topped with your own choice of fresh vegetables and low-fat ingredients. Look out for half-fat mozzarella cheese, which has only 10 g of fat per 100 g (3½ oz).

Five Veggie Pizza (V)

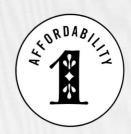

AFFORDABILITY 1

1 Put the flour, yeast, salt and oil in a bowl. Add the warm milk and water mixture and mix with a round-bladed knife to make a dough, adding a little more water if the dough feels dry and crumbly. Turn out on to a lightly floured surface and knead for 10 minutes until the dough is smooth and elastic. Put in a lightly oiled bowl, cover with clingfilm and leave to rise in a warm place for about 45 minutes until risen to about twice the size.

2 For the tomato sauce, put the tomatoes, tomato paste and garlic in a small saucepan and cook for 5 minutes until thickened.

3 For the topping, heat the oil in a non-stick frying pan and fry the fennel for 5 minutes, stirring. Add the courgette and red pepper and fry for 3 minutes, stirring. Tip in the spinach and turn with the cooked vegetables to lightly wilt. Season with salt and pepper.

4 Roll out the dough on a lightly floured surface until about 30 cm (12 inches) in diameter. Spread evenly with the tomato sauce and then scatter with the vegetables, spreading them to the edges. Arrange the mozzarella slices on top and sprinkle with the Parmesan-style or Cheddar-style cheese.

5 Bake in a preheated oven 230°C (450°F), Gas Mark 8, for 12 minutes or until the cheese is bubbling and golden. Serve with a mixed salad.

175 g (6 oz) malted grain bread flour, plus extra for dusting
1 teaspoon fast-action dried yeast
½ teaspoon salt
2 tablespoons olive oil, plus extra for greasing
100 ml (3½ fl oz) hand-hot mixed milk and water

Tomato sauce
200 g (7 oz) can chopped tomatoes
2 tablespoons sun-dried tomato paste
1 garlic clove, crushed

Topping
1 tablespoon olive oil
1 small fennel bulb, halved and thinly sliced
1 large courgette, about 200 g (7 oz), thinly sliced
1 red pepper, cored, deseeded and sliced
50 g (2 oz) spinach
125 g (4 oz) mozzarella cheese, thinly sliced
50 g (2 oz) Parmesan-style or mature Cheddar-style cheese, grated
salt and pepper

mixed salad, to serve

Calories per serving **458**
Serves **3**
Prep time **25 minutes, plus rising**
Cooking time **25 minutes**

PUMPKIN

& GOATS' CHEESE BAKE Ⓥ

1 Put the beetroot, pumpkin and onion into a roasting tin, drizzle with the oil and sprinkle with the fennel seeds and salt and pepper. Roast the vegetables in a preheated oven, 200°C (400°F), Gas Mark 6, for 20-25 minutes, turning once, until well browned and tender.

2 Cut the goats' cheeses in half and nestle each half among the roasted vegetables. Sprinkle the cheeses with a little salt and pepper and drizzle with some of the pan juices.

3 Return the dish to the oven for about 5 minutes, until the cheese is just beginning to melt. Sprinkle with rosemary and serve immediately.

VARIATION
For penne with beetroot and pumpkin, roast the vegetables as above for 20-25 minutes, omitting the fennel seeds. Cook 350 g (11½ oz) penne pasta in a saucepan of lightly salted boiling water according to the packet instructions, then drain, reserving one ladleful of the cooking water. Return the pasta to the pan and add the roasted vegetables, a handful of torn basil leaves and the cooking water. Omit the goats' cheese and rosemary. Cook over a high heat, stirring, for 30 seconds, then serve. Calories per serving 482

400 g (13 oz) raw beetroot, peeled and diced
625 g (1 ¼ lb) pumpkin or butternut squash, peeled, deseeded and cut into slightly larger dice
1 red onion, cut into wedges
2 tablespoons olive oil
2 teaspoons fennel seeds
2 small goats' cheeses, 100 g (3½ oz) each
salt and pepper
chopped rosemary, to garnish

Calories per serving **330**
Serves **4**
Prep time **20 minutes**
Cooking time **25-30 minutes**

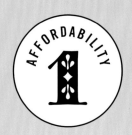

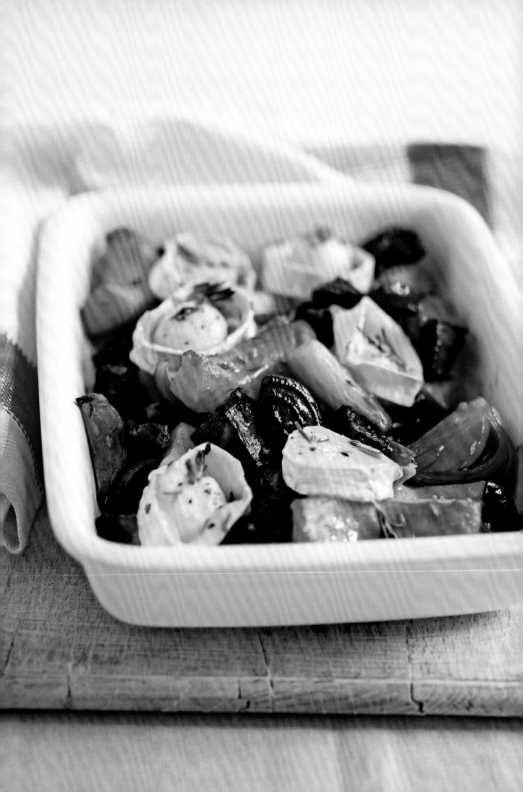

Mushroom Stroganoff

1 Melt the butter with the oil in a large, nonstick frying pan, add the onion and garlic and cook, stirring occasionally, until soft and starting to brown.

2 Add the mushrooms to the pan and cook, stirring occasionally, until soft and starting to brown. Stir in the mustard and crème fraîche and just heat through. Season to taste with salt and pepper, then serve immediately, garnished with the chopped parsley.

VARIATION

For mushroom soup with garlic croûtons, while the mushrooms are cooking, remove the crusts from 2 thick slices of day-old white bread and rub with 2 halved garlic cloves. Cut the bread into cubes. Fry the cubes of bread in a little vegetable oil in a nonstick frying pan, turning constantly, for 5 minutes or until browned all over and crisp. Drain on kitchen paper. After adding the mustard and crème fraîche to the mushroom mixture as above, add 400 ml (14 fl oz) hot Vegetable Stock (see page 244), then purée the mixture in a blender or food processor until smooth. Serve in bowls, topped with the croûtons and garnished with the chopped parsley. Calories per serving 273

1 tablespoon butter
2 tablespoons olive oil
1 onion, thinly sliced
4 garlic cloves, finely chopped
500 g (1 lb) chestnut mushrooms, trimmed and sliced
2 tablespoons wholegrain mustard
250 ml (8 fl oz) half-fat crème fraîche
salt and pepper
3 tablespoons chopped parsley, to garnish

Calories per serving **239**
Serves **4**
Prep time **10 minutes**
Cooking time **10 minutes**

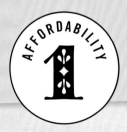

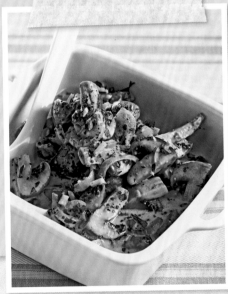

LEBANESE TOMATO & COURGETTE CURRY

Vegan

1 Heat the oil in a large, nonstick saucepan over a low heat. Add the onion and fry, stirring occasionally, for 10-12 minutes until soft and translucent. Add the courgettes and cook for a further 5-6 minutes, stirring occasionally.

2 Add the tomatoes (including the juice) and garlic and continue to cook over a medium heat for a further 20 minutes, stirring occasionally.

3 Stir in the chilli powder, turmeric and dried mint and cook for a few more minutes to allow the flavours to mingle. Season to taste with salt and pepper. Garnish with mint leaves and serve with boiled rice.

1 tablespoon light olive oil
1 large onion, finely chopped
4 courgettes, cut into 1 x 3.5 cm (½ x 1½ inch) batons
2 x 400 g (13 oz) cans whole plum tomatoes
2 garlic cloves, crushed
½ teaspoon chilli powder
¼ teaspoon ground turmeric
2 teaspoons dried mint
salt and pepper
mint leaves, to garnish
150 g (5 oz) Boiled Rice (see page 247) per person, to serve

Calories per serving **266**
Serves **4**
Prep time **10 minutes**
Cooking time **40-45 minutes**

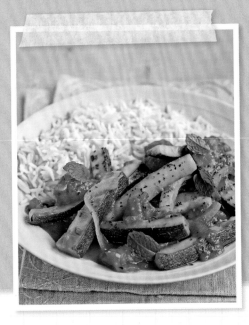

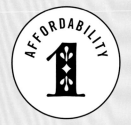
AFFORDABILITY 1

Sweet Alternatives

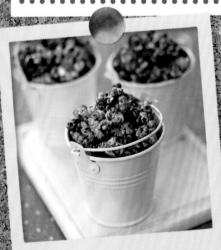

TOFFEE & CHOCOLATE POPCORN

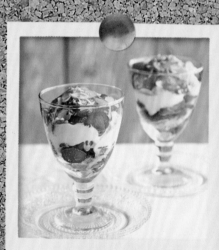

STRAWBERRY & ALMOND
LAYERED DESSERTS

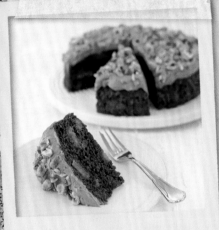

CHOCOLATE, COURGETTE & NUT CAKE

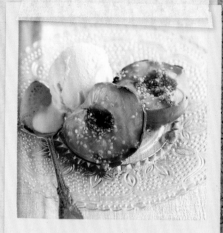

ROASTED HONEY PEACHES

LEMON DRIZZLE CAKE

1 Grease and line a 22 cm (8½ inch) square cake tin.

2 Put the eggs, caster sugar and salt in a large, heatproof bowl set over a saucepan of barely simmering water and beat with a hand-held electric whisk for 2–3 minutes or until the mixture triples in volume and thickens to the consistency of lightly whipped cream. Remove from the heat. Sift in the flour and baking powder, add the lemon rind and juice and drizzle the butter down the side of the bowl. Fold in gently.

3 Pour the mixture into the prepared tin. Bake in a preheated oven, 180°C (350°F), Gas Mark 4, for 20–25 minutes or until risen, golden and coming away from the sides of the tin.

4 Meanwhile, put all the syrup ingredients in a small saucepan and heat gently until the sugar dissolves, stirring. Increase the heat and boil rapidly, without stirring, for 4–5 minutes. Set aside to cool a little.

5 Leave the cake to cool in the tin for 5 minutes, then make holes over the surface with a skewer. Drizzle over two-thirds of the warm syrup (reserve the rest). Leave the cake to cool completely in the tin and absorb the syrup.

6 Turn the cake out of the tin and peel off the lining paper. Cut into squares or slices and serve each portion with about 1 heaped teaspoon of half-fat crème fraîche or soured cream and an extra drizzle of the remaining syrup.

VARIATION
For citrus drizzle cake with sorbet, make the cake as above, replacing the lemon rind and juice with the finely grated rind of 1 orange and 1 tablespoon orange juice. Serve topped with lemon sorbet.

100 g (3½ oz) butter, melted and cooled, plus extra for greasing
5 eggs
100 g (3½ oz) caster sugar
pinch of salt
125 g (4 oz) plain flour
1 teaspoon baking powder
finely grated rind of 1 lemon
1 tablespoon lemon juice

Syrup
250 g (8 oz) icing sugar, sifted
125 ml (4 fl oz) lemon juice
finely grated rind of 1 lemon
seeds scraped from 1 vanilla pod

half-fat crème fraîche or low-fat soured cream, to serve

Serves **8**
Prep time **20 minutes, plus cooling**
Cooking time **22–28 minutes**

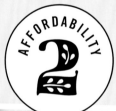

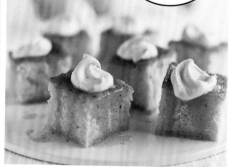

COURGETTE, LEMON & POPPY SEED CAKE

1 Grease and line a loaf tin with a capacity of about 500 g (1 lb) loaf tin.

2 Sift the flour and baking powder into a bowl. Beat the eggs in a separate mixing bowl with the oil, honey, sugar, poppy seeds and lemon rind and juice. Stir in the grated courgette. Add the flour and stir gently to mix.

3 Transfer the mixture to the prepared tin and level the surface. Bake in a preheated oven 160°C (325°F), Gas Mark 3, for 40–45 minutes or until risen and just firm to the touch. A skewer inserted into the centre should come out clean. Transfer to a wire rack to cool.

4 For the frosting, spoon the yogurt on to several sheets of kitchen paper. Place several more sheets on top and press firmly to squeeze out as much liquid as possible. Turn the yogurt into a bowl and stir in the lemon curd. Spread over the top of the cold cake. Serve in slices.

75 ml (3 fl oz) olive oil, plus extra
   for greasing
150 g (5 oz) spelt flour
1 teaspoon baking powder
2 eggs
50 ml (2 fl oz) clear honey
50 g (2 oz) caster sugar
2 tablespoons poppy seeds
finely grated rind and juice of
   1 lemon
100 g (3½ oz) courgette, grated

Frosting
125 ml (4 fl oz) 0%-fat Greek
   yogurt
2 tablespoons lemon curd

Serves **8**
Prep time **15 minutes, plus
cooling**
Cooking time **45 minutes**

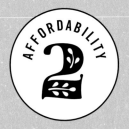

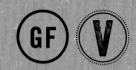

BLACKCURRANT
POLENTA MUG CAKE

1 Beat together the polenta, butter, honey and ground almonds in a 200 ml (7 fl oz) microwave-proof mug. Add the egg and beat together until well mixed. Microwave on full power for 1 minute.

2 Spoon the blackcurrants and blackcurrant preserve on top and stir in lightly so the polenta mixture is marbled with the fruit. Microwave on full power for 1 minute. Serve drizzled with extra honey.

2 tablespoons polenta
25 g (1 oz) slightly salted butter, softened
2 tablespoons clear honey, plus extra to drizzle
2 tablespoons ground almonds
1 egg
2 tablespoons blackcurrants, topped and tailed
1 tablespoon blackcurrant preserve

Serves **1**
Prep time **5 minutes**
Cooking time **2 minutes**

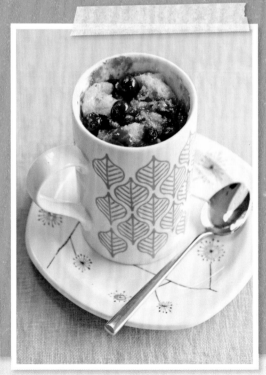

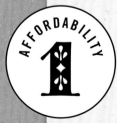

SPICED PASSION
MUG CAKE

1 Put the honey, butter, egg, flour and ginger in a 350 ml (12 fl oz) microwave-proof mug and beat together until well mixed. Add the carrot and pineapple and mix well.

2 Microwave on full power for 2 minutes or until just firm to touch and a cocktail stick inserted into the centre comes out clean. Serve topped with the cream cheese and drizzled with the ginger syrup.

2 tablespoons clear honey
25 g (1 oz) slightly salted butter, softened
1 egg
3 tablespoons self-raising flour
2.5 cm (1 inch) piece of preserved stem ginger in syrup, drained and chopped
5 cm (2 inch) piece of carrot, finely grated
½ fresh or canned pineapple ring, chopped
1 tablespoon cream cheese
1 tablespoon preserved stem ginger syrup, to drizzle

Serves **1**
Prep time **5 minutes**
Cooking time **2 minutes**

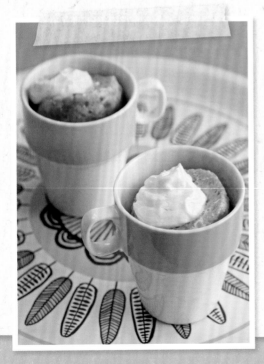

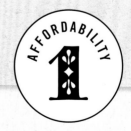

AFFORDABILITY
1

Chocolate, COURGETTE & NUT CAKE

1 Grease and line a 20 cm (8 inch) round, deep, loose-bottomed cake tin.

2 Place the courgettes in a sieve and squeeze out any excess liquid. Beat together the eggs, oil, orange rind and juice and sugar in a large bowl. Sift in the flour, cocoa powder, bicarbonate of soda and baking powder and beat to combine. Fold in the courgettes and apricots, then spoon the mixture into the prepared tin and level the surface.

3 Bake in a preheated oven, 180°C (350°F), Gas Mark 4, for 40 minutes until risen and firm to the touch. Let cool in the tin for 5 minutes. Turn out on to a wire rack and leave to cool completely.

4 For the topping, beat together the cream cheese and chocolate hazelnut spread in a bowl, then spread over the top of the cake. Sprinkle over the chopped hazelnuts. Serve in slices.

100 ml (3½ fl oz) vegetable oil, plus extra for greasing
250 g (8 oz) courgettes, coarsely grated
2 eggs
finely grated rind and juice of 1 orange
125 g (4 oz) caster sugar
225 g (7½ oz) self-raising flour
2 tablespoons cocoa powder
½ teaspoon bicarbonate of soda
½ teaspoon baking powder
50 g (2 oz) ready-to-eat dried apricots, chopped

Topping
200 g (7 oz) cream cheese
2 tablespoons vegetarian-friendly chocolate hazelnut spread
1 tablespoon hazelnuts, toasted and chopped

Serves **12**
Prep time **20 minutes, plus cooling**
Cooking time **40 minutes**

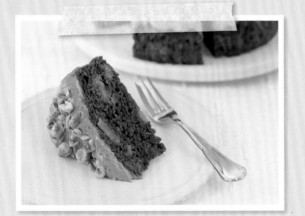

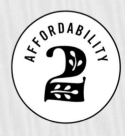

GLUTEN-FREE
COCONUT & MANGO CAKE

THIS DELICIOUS TROPICAL-INSPIRED CAKE IS GREAT FOR SUMMER EATING WITH A BUNCH OF FRIENDS.

1 Grease and line a 23 cm (9 inch) round, deep, loose-bottomed cake tin.

2 Place the butter and brown sugar in a large bowl and beat together until light and fluffy, then beat in the egg yolks, buttermilk, polenta, rice flour, baking powder, coconut milk powder and desiccated coconut. Whisk the egg whites in a separate large, clean bowl until they form soft peaks, then fold into the cake mixture with the puréed mango.

3 Spoon the mixture into the prepared tin, level the surface, then bake in a preheated oven, 200°C (400°F) Gas Mark 6, for 45-50 minutes until golden and firm to the touch. Let cool in the tin for 5 minutes. Transfer to a wire rack to cool completely.

4 When the cake is cold, slice it in half horizontally. Place the filling ingredients in a bowl and mix together until combined. Use half of the filling to sandwich the cake together, then spread the remaining mixture over the top. Serve in slices.

100 g (3½ oz) butter, softened, plus extra for greasing
100 g (3½ oz) soft light brown sugar
4 eggs, separated
400 ml (14 fl oz) buttermilk
200 g (7 oz) polenta
200 g (7 oz) rice flour
2 teaspoons gluten-free baking powder
50 g (2 oz) coconut milk powder
50 g (2 oz) desiccated coconut
1 ripe mango, peeled, stoned and flesh puréed

Filling
250 g (8 oz) mascarpone cheese
1 ripe mango, peeled, stoned and finely chopped
2 tablespoons icing sugar

Serves **12**
Prep time **20 minutes, plus cooling**
Cooking time **45-50 minutes**

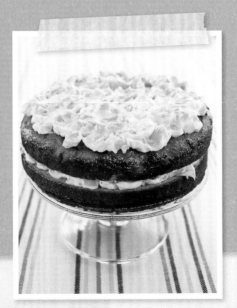

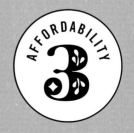

EASY ALMOND MACAROONS

1 Line a large baking sheet with nonstick baking paper.

2 Whisk the egg whites in a clean bowl with a hand-held electric whisk until soft peaks form. Gradually whisk in the sugar, a spoonful at a time, until thick and glossy. Fold in the ground almonds until combined.

3 Drop dessertspoonfuls of the mixture, slightly apart, on to the prepared baking sheet. Press an almond on top of each.

4 Bake in a preheated oven, 180°C (350°F), Gas Mark 4, for about 15 minutes until the biscuits are pale golden and just crisp. Leave on the paper to cool for 5 minutes, then transfer to a wire rack to cool completely before serving.

VARIATION

For scribbled chocolate macaroons, make the macaroons as above, replacing 20 g (¾ oz) of the ground almonds with 20 g (¾ oz) cocoa powder and omitting the whole almonds. Heat 50 g (2 oz) plain dark or milk chocolate, evenly chopped, in a microwave-proof mug in a microwave in two or three 30-second bursts, stirring inbetween, until melted. Drizzle over the cooled biscuits with a teaspoon. Leave the chocolate to set before serving.

2 egg whites
100 g (3½ oz) golden caster sugar
100 g (3½ oz) ground almonds
blanched whole almonds, to decorate

Makes about **15**
Prep time **15 minutes, plus cooling**
Cooking time **15 minutes**

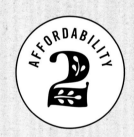

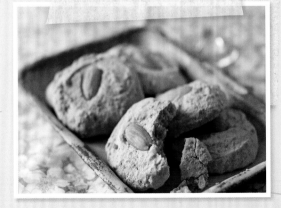

CHOCOLATE PEANUT COOKIES (V)

1 Line a large baking sheet with nonstick baking paper.

2 Combine the flour, bicarbonate of soda and sugar in a bowl. Add the peanut butter, honey, oil and chocolate and mix to form a thick paste.

3 Take spoonfuls of the mixture and roll between the palms of your hands into a ball, each about the size of a whole walnut. Space well apart on the prepared baking sheet.

4 Bake in a preheated oven 190°C (375°F), Gas Mark 5, for 10 minutes until the cookies have risen and turned golden. Leave on the baking sheet for 2 minutes to firm up, then transfer to a wire rack to cool completely.

100 g (3 ½ oz) rice flour
1 teaspoon bicarbonate of soda
50 g (2 oz) light muscovado sugar
200 g (7 oz) crunchy peanut butter
50 g (2 oz) clear honey
2 tablespoons mild olive oil or vegetable oil
75 g (3 oz) plain dark chocolate, chopped

Makes **20**
Prep time **10 minutes, plus cooling**
Cooking time **10 minutes**

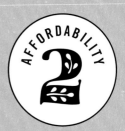

AFFORDABILITY
2

BUG BUSTING

Unfortunately, student living goes hand in hand with getting ill. Living in close proximity to other people harbouring a bunch of germs, combined with burning the candle at both ends, is a sure-fire way to end up sick in bed. Common coughs and colds, the dreaded flu and other contagious illnesses are all part and parcel of leaving home. But there are certain steps you can take to minimize your chances of festering in a cold sweat in your room without your mum to mop your brow.

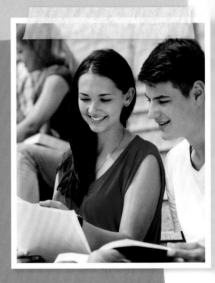

SLEEP

While it's tempting to let your shut-eye suffer as you try to keep up with work and a packed social life, a lack of sleep will soon see you getting run down and more prone to picking up infections. Sleep deprivation can have a big impact on your immune system and you'll be more likely to pick up illnesses and take longer to recover if you haven't been getting the ideal 7–9 hours a night.

DON'T STRESS OUT

The stereotype of the lazy student is seriously outdated and it's stress that we need to worry about these days. With the pressure piled on for essays and exams, and working and living independently, it's no surprise that students feel a bit strung out. But stress can have an adverse effect on your health and lead to illness, so it's important to manage stress before it takes over your life.

HYGIENE

Germs love nothing more than poor hygiene so don't
encourage them – wash your hands with antibacterial
soap, keep bathrooms and kitchens clean, and be
extra careful with food prep. It also makes sense to
steer clear of your mates when they're harbouring an
unpleasant illness.

EXERCISE

Regular exercise can help to build a
healthy immune system by promoting
good circulation.

HEALTHY EATING

It goes without saying that a
balanced, healthy diet will boost
your body's natural defences against
viruses and will help you to fight
infection if you do become ill.

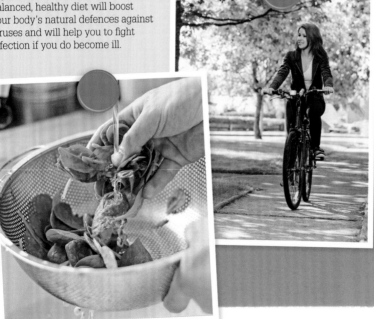

CRANBERRY & HAZELNUT COOKIES Ⓥ

1 Line 2 large baking sheets with greaseproof or nonstick baking paper.

2 Beat together the butter, sugars, egg and vanilla essence in a large bowl until smooth. Stir in the flour and oats, then the cranberries and hazelnuts.

3 Place teaspoonfuls of the mixture on to the prepared baking sheets, leaving space between each one, then flatten them slightly with the back of a fork.

4 Bake in a preheated oven, 180°C (350°F), Gas Mark 4, for about 5-6 minutes until lightly browned. Let cool for 2-3 minutes. Transfer to a wire rack and leave to cool completely.

VARIATION
For plain dark chocolate and ginger cookies, prepare the mixture as above, omitting the dried cranberries and hazelnuts. Replace them with 40 g (1 ½ oz) plain dark chocolate chips or chunks and 2 pieces of drained, chopped preserved stem ginger (or ½ teaspoon peeled and grated fresh root ginger). Stir together, then bake and cool as above.

50 g (2 oz) unsalted butter, softened
40 g (1 ½ oz) granulated sugar
25 g (1 oz) soft light brown sugar
1 egg, beaten
few drops of vanilla essence
150 g (5 oz) self-raising flour, sifted
50 g (2 oz) rolled oats
50 g (2 oz) dried cranberries
40 g (1½ oz) hazelnuts, toasted and chopped

Makes **30**
Prep time **10 minutes, plus cooling**
Cooking time **6 minutes**

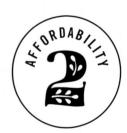

TOFFEE & CHOCOLATE
POPCORN

1 Put the popping corn in a large bowl. Cover the bowl
with a vented food cover (or greaseproof paper held in
place with an elastic band with slits cut into it).
Microwave on full power for 4 minutes. Alternatively,
cook in a pan with a lid on the hob, over a medium heat,
for a few minutes, shaking the pan occasionally to avoid
burning the kernels, until popping rapidly then remove
from the heat and leave until the popping stops.

2 Meanwhile, gently heat the butter, muscovado sugar and
cocoa powder together in a pan, stirring until the sugar
has dissolved and the butter has melted. Stir the warm
popcorn into the mixture and serve.

VARIATION
For toffee, marshmallow and nut popcorn, omit the muscovado
sugar and cocoa powder. Microwave the popping corn as
above, then gently heat 150 g (5 oz) chewy toffees,
125 g (4 oz) butter, 125 g (4 oz) marshmallows and
50 g (2 oz) plain dark chocolate in a pan until
melted and combined. Serve as above.

125 g (4 oz) popping corn
250 g (8 oz) butter
250 g (8 oz) light muscovado
   sugar
2 tablespoons cocoa powder

Serves **12 as a snack**
Prep time **1 minutes**
Cooking time **4 minutes**

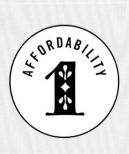

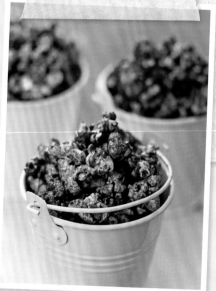

MANGO & PASSION FRUIT
TRIFLE

1 Break each sponge finger into 4 pieces and divide between 2 glasses. Mix the yogurt and crème fraîche together in a bowl.

2 Halve the passion fruit and scoop out the pulpy seeds. Spoon two-thirds of the seeds over the sponge fingers, then add half of the mango pieces.

3 Spoon half of the crème fraîche mixture over the fruit, then top with the remaining mango. Spoon over the remaining crème fraîche mixture and top with the remaining passion fruit seeds. Chill in the refrigerator for 1 hour before serving.

2 sponge fingers
75 ml (3 fl oz) 0%-fat Greek yogurt
100 ml (3 ½ fl oz) half-fat crème fraîche
2 passion fruit
½ ripe mango, peeled, stoned and diced

Serves **2**
Prep time **15 minutes, plus chilling**

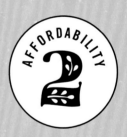

BAKED STRAWBERRIES & MERINGUE Ⓥ

1 Line 4 individual tart tins or ramekins with nonstick baking paper.

2 Whisk the egg whites in a bowl until they form stiff peaks, then beat in the sugar, a spoonful at a time, making sure the sugar is incorporated between additions. Fold in the cornflour, vinegar and vanilla extract until combined.

3 Spoon the mixture into the prepared tart tins or ramekins and cook in a preheated oven, 120°C (250°F), Gas Mark ½, for 2½ hours. Place the strawberries in an ovenproof dish and bake with the meringues for the last hour of the cooking time.

4 Spoon the baked strawberries and any cooking juices over the meringues to serve.

VARIATION
For baked nectarines with orange meringues, add the finely grated rind of 1 orange to the meringue mixture with the cornflour. Cut 2 peeled and stoned nectarines into thin slices and place in an ovenproof dish. Sprinkle with 2 tablespoons sugar and 1 tablespoon orange juice, then bake for 45 minutes with the meringues. Serve the fruit over the meringues.

3 egg whites
150 g (5 oz) light muscovado sugar
1 tablespoon cornflour
1 teaspoon white vinegar
1 teaspoon vanilla extract
250 g (8 oz) strawberries, hulled and sliced

Serves **4**
Prep time **15 minutes**
Cooking time **2½ hours**

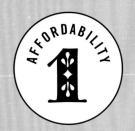

AFFORDABILITY
1

ROASTED HONEY PEACHES

1 Spoon the honey into a small saucepan. Scrape the seeds from the vanilla pod and add the seeds and pod to the pan. Heat gently, stirring occasionally for 1-2 minutes. Stir in the sesame seeds.

2 Place the peaches cut side down in a roasting tin and pour over the honey mixture. Bake in a preheated oven, 180°C (350°F), Gas Mark 4, for 20-25 minutes until the peaches are soft. Baste a couple of times with the juices during cooking.

3 Serve the baked peaches warm with vanilla ice cream or crème fraîche, if liked.

2 tablespoons orange blossom honey
1 vanilla pod, split in half lengthways
2-3 teaspoons sesame seeds
4 peaches, halved and stoned
vanilla ice cream or half-fat crème fraîche, to serve (optional)

Serves **4**
Prep time **10 minutes**
Cooking time **25-30 minutes**

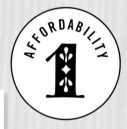

AFFORDABILITY 1

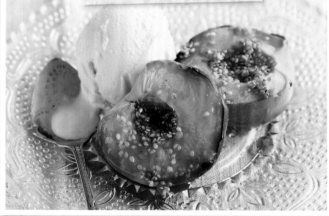

BERRY & MINT COMPOTE

1 Place the fruit, cinnamon stick and orange rind and juice in a small saucepan and simmer gently for 12–15 minutes.

2 Remove the cinnamon stick and leave the compote to cool for 3–4 minutes, then stir in the mint.

3 Serve with dollops of natural yogurt, if liked.

450 g (14½ oz) mixed fruit, such as strawberries, blackberries, raspberries and halved and stoned plums
1 cinnamon stick
finely grated rind and juice of 1 orange
8 mint leaves, shredded
natural yogurt, to serve (optional)

Serves **4**
Prep time **10 minutes, plus cooling**
Cooking time **15 minutes**

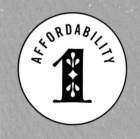

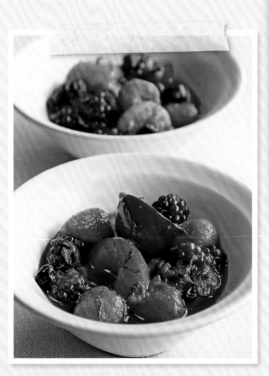

Instant
APPLE CRUMBLES

1 Place the apples in a saucepan with the butter, caster sugar, lemon juice and water. Cover and simmer for 8-10 minutes, until softened. Remove from the heat.

2 For the crumble, melt the butter in a frying pan, add the breadcrumbs and stir-fry over medium heat until light golden, then add the pumpkin seeds and stir-fry for a further 1 minute. Remove from the heat and stir in the brown sugar.

3 Spoon the apple mixture into bowls, sprinkle with the crumble and serve.

VARIATION
For instant pear and chocolate crumbles, peel, core and slice 1 kg (2 lb) pears and cook them with the butter, caster sugar and water as above, adding ½ teaspoon ground ginger instead of the lemon juice. Prepare the crumble as above, replacing the pumpkin seeds with 50 g (2 oz) roughly chopped plain dark chocolate. Cook and serve as above.

1 kg (2 lb) cooking apples, such as Bramley, peeled, cored and thickly sliced
25 g (1 oz) butter
2 tablespoons caster sugar
1 tablespoon lemon juice
2 tablespoons water

Crumble
50 g (2 oz) butter
75 g (3 oz) fresh wholemeal breadcrumbs
25 g (1 oz) pumpkin seeds
2 tablespoons soft brown sugar

Serves **4**
Prep time **10 minutes**
Cooking time **13 minutes**

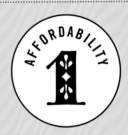

AFFORDABILITY
1

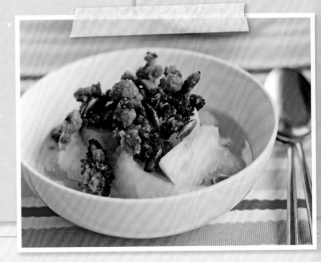

STRAWBERRY & ALMOND LAYERED DESSERTS

1   Place the flaked almonds and coconut on a baking sheet and cook under a preheated medium-hot grill for 3–4 minutes until golden. Give the tray a little shake at least once to ensure the almonds are lightly toasted on both sides. Leave to cool.

2   Spoon half of the almond and coconut mixture into 4 glasses. Top with half of the sliced strawberries, then all of the yogurt.

3   Top with the remaining strawberries, then the remaining almond and coconut mixture. Spoon over the honey and serve.

4 tablespoons flaked almonds
4 tablespoons desiccated coconut
300 g (10 oz) strawberries, hulled and sliced
250 ml (8 fl oz) natural yogurt
4 teaspoons clear honey

Serves **4**
Prep time **10 minutes, plus cooling**
Cooking time **3–4 minutes**

AFFORDABILITY 1

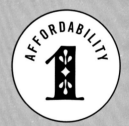

LEMON & SULTANA RICE PUDDING (V)

1 Scrape the seeds from the vanilla pod and add the seeds and pod to a saucepan with the rice, milk, sultanas and lemon rind.

2 Bring to the boil, then reduce the heat and simmer for 15-18 minutes, stirring occasionally, until the rice is swollen and soft. Stir in the sugar to taste and leave to cool for 10 minutes.

3 Remove the vanilla pod from the rice, then stir in the yogurt. Serve sprinkled with a little nutmeg.

1 vanilla pod, split in half lengthways
175 g (6 oz) short-grain rice
750 ml (1¼ pints) milk
2 tablespoons sultanas
finely grated rind of 2 lemons
2 teaspoons caster sugar, or to taste
150 ml (¼ pint) thick natural yogurt
ground or freshly grated nutmeg, to serve

Serves **8**
Prep time **10 minutes, plus cooling**
Cooking time **20 minutes**

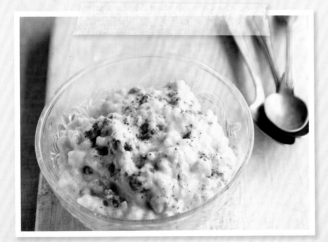

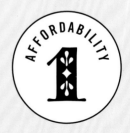

AFFORDABILITY 1

Warm Chocolate
FROMAGE FRAIS

1 Melt the chocolate in a heatproof bowl set over a saucepan of barely simmering water, then remove from the heat. Add the fromage frais and vanilla extract and quickly stir together.

2 Divide the chocolate fromage frais between 6 little pots or glasses and serve immediately.

VARIATION
For warm cappuccino fromage frais, melt the plain dark chocolate with 2 tablespoons very strong (brewed) espresso coffee and then add the fat-free fromage frais. Divide between 6 espresso cups, finishing each with 1 teaspoon fromage frais and a dusting of cocoa powder.

300 g (10 oz) plain dark chocolate, broken into squares
500 g (1 lb) fat-free fromage frais
1 teaspoon vanilla extract

Serves **6**
Prep time **5 minutes**
Cooking time **5 minutes**

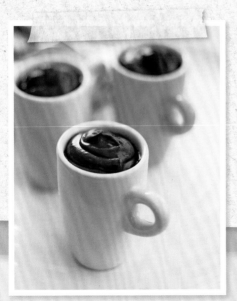

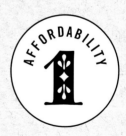
AFFORDABILITY
1

WHITE *Chocolate* MOUSSE

1. Put the chocolate and milk in a heatproof bowl and melt over a saucepan of barely simmering water.

2. To release the cardamom seeds, crush the pods using a pestle and mortar. Discard the pods and crush the seeds finely. Place the crushed cardamom seeds and the tofu in a blender or food processor with half of the sugar, then blend well to make a smooth paste. Turn the mixture into a large bowl.

3. Whisk the egg white in a separate clean bowl, until it forms soft peaks. Gradually whisk in the remaining sugar.

4. Beat the melted chocolate mixture into the tofu until completely combined. Using a large metal spoon, fold in the whisked egg white.

5. Spoon the mousse into small coffee cups or glasses and chill in the refrigerator for at least 1 hour before serving. Serve topped with spoonfuls of crème fraîche or yogurt and a light dusting of cocoa powder.

VARIATION

For white chocolate and amaretto pots, make the mousse mixture as above, omitting the cardamom and adding 2 tablespoons Amaretto liqueur when blending the tofu. Complete the recipe and chill as above. Serve with fresh raspberries instead of the crème fraîche or yogurt and cocoa powder.

200 g (7 oz) white chocolate, chopped
4 tablespoons milk
12 cardamom pods
200 g (7 oz) silken tofu
50 g (2 oz) caster sugar
1 egg white
half-fat crème fraîche or natural yogurt, to serve
cocoa powder, for dusting

Serves **6-8**
Prep time **15 minutes, plus chilling**
Cooking time **5 minutes**

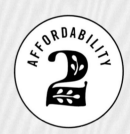

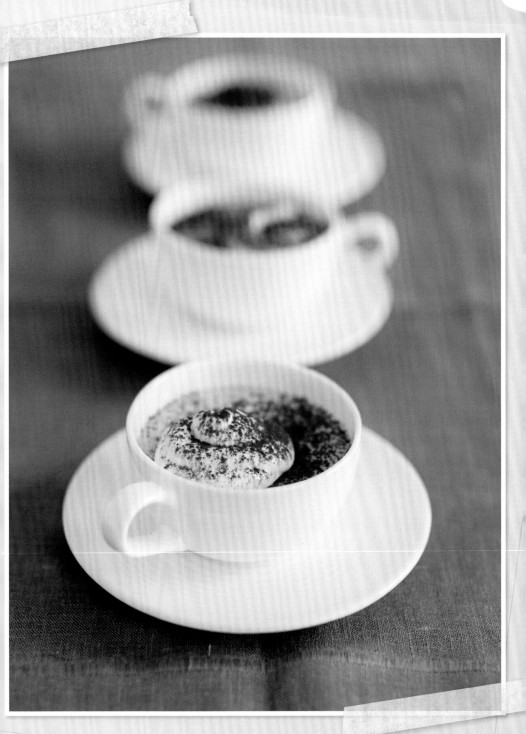

Cidered Apple Jellies

1 Put the apples, cider, 150 ml (¼ pint) water, sugar and the rind of 1 of the lemons into a saucepan. Cover and simmer for 15 minutes until the apples are soft.

2 Meanwhile, put the remaining 4 tablespoons of water into a small bowl and sprinkle over the gelatine, making sure that all the powder is absorbed by the water. Set aside.

3 Add the gelatine to the hot apples and stir until completely dissolved. Purée the apple mixture in a blender or food processor until smooth, then pour into 6 teacups or glasses. Leave to cool, then chill in the refrigerator for 4–5 hours until completely set.

4 When you are ready to serve, whip the cream in a bowl until it forms soft peaks. Spoon the cream over the jellies and sprinkle with the remaining lemon rind, then serve.

VARIATION

For cidered apple granita, omit the gelatine and pour the puréed apple mixture into a shallow dish so that the mixture is about 2.5 cm (1 inch) deep or less. Freeze for about 2 hours until mushy around the edges, then beat with a fork. Freeze for a further 2 hours, beating the granita at 30-minute intervals until it becomes the texture of crushed ice. Freeze until ready to serve, then scoop into small glasses.

1 kg (2 lb) cooking apples, peeled, cored and sliced
300 ml (½ pint) cider
150 ml (¼ pint) water, plus 4 tablespoons
75 g (3 oz) caster sugar
finely grated rind of 2 lemons
4 teaspoons powdered gelatine
150 ml (¼ pint) double cream

Serves **6**
Prep time **20 minutes, plus cooling and chilling**
Cooking time **15 minutes**

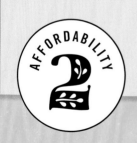

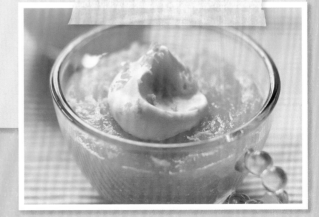

Griddled Bananas
WITH BLUEBERRIES

V

1 Heat a ridged griddle pan over a medium-high heat, add the bananas and griddle for 8-10 minutes or until the skins are beginning to blacken, turning occasionally.

2 Transfer the bananas to serving dishes and, using a sharp knife, cut open lengthways. Spoon over the yogurt and sprinkle with the oatmeal or oats and blueberries. Serve immediately, drizzled with about 1 teaspoon honey per banana.

VARIATION
For oatmeal, ginger and sultana yogurt, mix 1/2 teaspoon ground ginger with the yogurt in a bowl. Sprinkle with 2-4 tablespoons soft dark brown sugar, according to taste, the oatmeal and 4 tablespoons sultanas. Leave to stand for 5 minutes before serving.

4 bananas, unpeeled
8 tablespoons 0%-fat Greek yogurt
4 tablespoons oatmeal or fine porridge oats
125 g (4 oz) blueberries
clear honey, to serve

Serves **4**
Prep time **5 minutes**
Cooking time **8-10 minutes, plus standing**

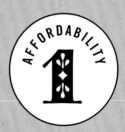

AFFORDABILITY 1

Back to Basics

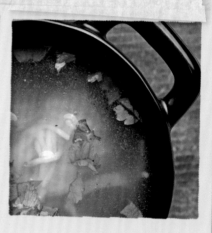

CHICKEN STOCK

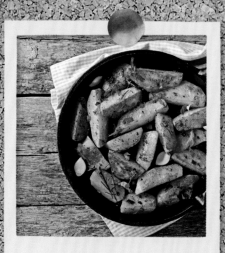

PERFECT ROAST POTATOES

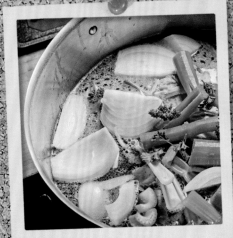

VEGETABLE STOCK

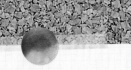

FRESH TOMATO SAUCE

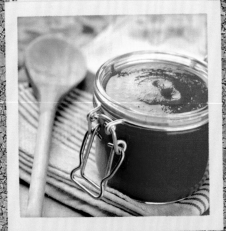

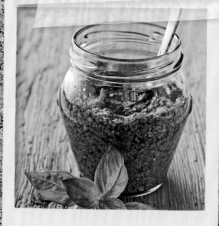

PESTO

Vegetable Stock

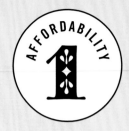

THE VEGETABLES CAN VARY BUT MAKE SURE YOU
INCLUDE SOME ONION AND OMIT VEGETABLES WITH
STRONG FLAVOURS AND STARCHY ONES LIKE POTATOES.
FOR A DARK STOCK, LEAVE THE SKINS ON THE ONIONS
AND USE PLENTY OF MUSHROOMS.

1 Heat the oil in a large, heavy-based saucepan and gently fry
all the vegetables for 5 minutes.

2 Add the water, bouquet garni and peppercorns, bring slowly
to the boil. Reduce the heat and simmer the stock very
gently for 40 minutes, skimming the surface from time to
time if necessary.

3 Strain the stock through a large sieve, preferably a conical
one. Don't squeeze the juice out of the vegetables or the
stock will be cloudy. Leave the stock to cool completely,
then chill.

1 tablespoon sunflower oil
2 onions, roughly chopped
2 carrots, roughly chopped
2 celery sticks, roughly chopped
500 g (1 lb) mixture of other
   prepared fresh vegetables (such
   as parsnips, fennel, leeks,
   courgettes, mushrooms and
   tomatoes)
1.5 litres (2½ pints) water
1 bouquet garni
1 teaspoon black peppercorns

Makes about **1 litre (1¾ pints)**
Prep time **10 minutes**
Cooking time **45 minutes**

CHICKEN STOCK

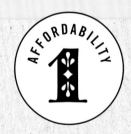

IDEALLY CHICKEN STOCK IS MADE USING A RAW
CARCASS, BUT A COOKED CARCASS ALSO MAKES
A WELL-FLAVOURED STOCK, IF A LITTLE CLOUDY.

1 Put the chicken carcass, giblets, onion, celery, bouquet
garni or bay leaves and peppercorns into a large, heavy-
based saucepan with the water.

2 Bring slowly to the boil. Reduce the heat and simmer the
stock very gently for 1½ hours, skimming the surface from
time to time if necessary.

3 Strain the stock through a large sieve, preferably a conical
one. Leave the stock to cool completely, then chill.

1 large chicken carcass, plus any
   trimmings
giblets, except the liver, if available
1 onion, quartered
1 celery stick, roughly chopped
1 bouquet garni or 3 bay leaves
1 teaspoon black peppercorns
1.8 litres (3 pints) cold water

Makes about **1 litre (1¾ pints)**
Prep time **10 minutes**
Cooking time **1½ hours**

GRAVY

GOOD-QUALITY CUTS OF ROASTED MEAT OR POULTRY PROVIDE DELICIOUS FATS AND JUICES FOR A WELL-FLAVOURED GRAVY. AFTER ROASTING, LIFT THE MEAT FROM THE TRAY, COVER IT LOOSELY WITH KITCHEN FOIL AND MAKE THE GRAVY WHILE THE MEAT STANDS.

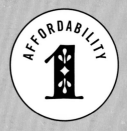

1 Tilt the flameproof roasting tin and skim off the fat from the surface with a large serving spoon until you are left with the pan juices and just a thin layer of fat.

2 Over a medium heat on the hob, sprinkle the flour into the tin and stir with a wooden spoon, scraping up all the residue, particularly from around the edges of the tin.

3 Gradually pour the liquid into the tin, stirring well until the gravy is thick and glossy. Let the mixture bubble, then check the seasoning, adding a little salt and pepper if necessary.

pan juices from roasted meat
1 tablespoon plain flour (less for a thin gravy)
300–400 ml (10–14 fl oz) liquid (this could be water, drained from the accompanying vegetables; stock; half stock and half water; or half wine and half water)
salt and pepper

Makes about **600 ml (1 pint)**
Cooking time **5 minutes**

OMELETTE Ⓥ

1 Break the eggs into a bowl and beat lightly with a balloon whisk. Whisk in the water and season well with salt and pepper. Do not over-beat because this will ruin the texture of the finished omelette.

2 Set a small frying pan over a gentle heat and, when it is hot, add the butter. Tip the pan so that the entire inner surface is coated with butter. When the butter is foaming, but not browned, tip in the beaten eggs.

3 Leave for a few seconds then, using a spatula, draw the mixture away from the edge of the pan into the centre, allowing the eggs to run to the sides. Repeat the process twice more, by which time the eggs should have set. Cook for a further 30 seconds until the underside is golden and top still slightly runny and creamy.

4 Tilt the pan and, with the spatula, carefully turn the omelette on to a plate, folding it in half in the process.

2 eggs
1 tablespoon water
15 g (½ oz) butter
salt and pepper

Serves **1**
Prep time **2 minutes**
Cooking time **3-4 minutes**

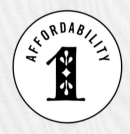

STUDENT TIP

Grow your own… cooking herbs that is! You don't need a big garden — or any outside space for that matter (a windowsill will do) — to grow some essential herbs. For the price of a few plastic containers and packets of seeds, you could have your own collection of basil, parsley and mint, ready to add another level to boring soups and sauces. Herbs also freeze well and you can use directly from frozen — so no more waste.

HOW TO MAKE *Perfect* ROAST POTATOES

NO ROAST DINNER IS COMPLETE WITHOUT POTATOES, SO IF YOU'VE EVER WONDERED HOW TO MAKE SCRUMPTIOUS ROASTIES – LOOK NO FURTHER!

1 Peel and cut potatoes into even-sized pieces. Parboil in a saucepan of lightly salted boiling water for 10 minutes, then drain well. Shake them after draining to rough up the edges slightly.

2 Heat a roasting tin containing lard (or a good glug of sunflower oil for veggies and vegans) in a preheated oven, 220°C (425°F), Gas Mark 7, for about 5 minutes or until the lard or oil is very hot. Carefully place the potatoes in it, turning them over in the oil and then lightly sprinkle with sea salt.

3 Roast on the top shelf in the oven for 40 minutes, turning every now and then, until golden and crispy. Serve.

potatoes
lard or sunflower oil
sea salt

Serves **4-6**
Prep time **5 minutes**
Cooking time **55 minutes**

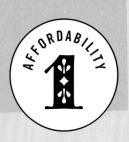

BOILED RICE

1 Put the rice in a sieve and wash it under running warm water, rubbing the grains together between your hands to get rid of any excess starch.

2 Put the rice into a saucepan and add the stock. Set the pan on the smallest ring on the hob and bring it to the boil. Give it a quick stir, then reduce the heat to a simmer. Cover with a lid and leave to cook for 15 minutes.

3 Turn off the heat and allow the rice to steam with the lid on for another 20 minutes. Don't be tempted to lift the lid to check what's going on.

4 To serve, fluff up the grains of rice with a spoon or fork.

350 g (11 ½ oz) Thai jasmine or long-grain rice
300 ml (½ pint) Vegetable or Chicken Stock (see pages 244)

Serves **4**
Prep time **5 minutes**
Cooking time **20 minutes, plus 20 minutes standing**

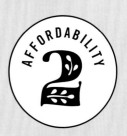

PESTO ⓥ

MAKING PESTO TRADITIONALLY USING A PESTLE AND MORTAR FILLS THE AIR WITH THE
WONDERFUL FRAGRANCE OF CRUSHED BASIL LEAVES, BUT IS MORE TIME-CONSUMING
THAN THE QUICK AND EASY FOOD PROCESSOR METHOD USED HERE. FRESHLY-MADE
PESTO HAS NUMEROUS USES, MOST COMMONLY AS A PASTA SAUCE BUT ALSO TO
FLAVOUR SOUPS, STEWS AND RISOTTOS.

1 Tear the basil into pieces and put it into a blender or food
   processor with the pine nuts, cheese and garlic.

2 Process lightly until the nuts are broken into small pieces,
   scraping the mixture down from the sides of the bowl if
   necessary.

3 Add the oil and a little salt and pepper and blend to form
   a thick paste. Stir into freshly cooked pasta or turn into a
   bowl, cover and refrigerate. It can be kept, covered, for up
   to 5 days.

50 g (2 oz) fresh basil, including
  stalks
50 g (2 oz) pine nuts
65 g (2 ½ oz) grated Parmesan-
  style cheese
2 garlic cloves, chopped
125 ml (4 fl oz) olive oil
salt and pepper

Serves **4**
Prep time **5 minutes**

VARIATION

To make red pesto, drain 125 g (4 oz) sun-dried tomatoes in oil,
chop them into small pieces and add to the food processor
instead of the basil.

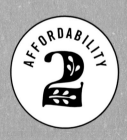

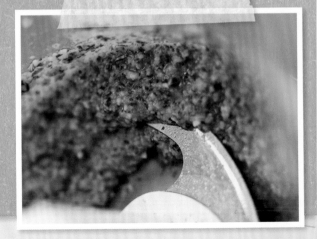

FRESH TOMATO SAUCE

THE RICH, FRUITY FLAVOUR OF THIS SAUCE IS ONE OF THE BEST AND MOST USEFUL IN PASTA DISHES. USE IT AS IT IS OR ADD OTHER INGREDIENTS, SUCH AS CAPERS, ANCHOVIES, COOKED PANCETTA OR TORN BASIL.

1 Put the tomatoes in a heatproof bowl, cover with boiling water and leave for about 2 minutes or until the skins start to split. Pour away the water. Skin and roughly chop the tomatoes.

2 Heat the oil in a large, heavy-based saucepan and gently fry the onion for 5 minutes or until softened but not browned. Add the garlic and fry for a further 1 minute.

3 Add the tomatoes and cook, stirring frequently, for 20-25 minutes or until the sauce is thickened and pulpy.

4 Stir in the oregano and season to taste with salt and pepper. If the sauce is very sharp, add a sprinkling of caster sugar, if liked.

TIP
This is a good sauce to make in large quantities if you have a glut of tomatoes and can be frozen in small polythene freezer bags or plastic containers.

VARIATION
Canned tomatoes make a good alternative if the only fresh ones available don't look very appetizing. Substitute two 400 g (13 oz) cans of chopped tomatoes and cook until pulpy.

1 kg (2 lb) very ripe, full-flavoured tomatoes
100 ml (3 ½ fl oz) olive oil
1 onion, finely chopped
2 garlic cloves, crushed
2 tablespoons chopped oregano
sprinkling of caster sugar (optional)
salt and pepper

Makes **750 ml (1¼ pints)**
Prep time **15 minutes**
Cooking time **30 minutes**

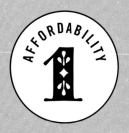

BÉCHAMEL SAUCE

THIS CREAMY WHITE SAUCE IS USED AS A TOPPING FOR LASAGNE AND OTHER PASTA BAKES. IF THERE'S ADDITIONAL CREAM IN THE PASTA RECIPE YOU MIGHT PREFER TO USE EXTRA MILK INSTEAD.

1 Melt the butter over a medium heat in a small, heavy-based saucepan. Stir in the flour and cook gently for 1-2 minutes, stirring to make a smooth paste.

2 Remove the pan from the heat and add the milk (very gradually to avoid lumps forming), continuously whisking or beating well with a wooden spoon. When all the milk is combined you should have a smooth sauce.

3 Stir in the cream or additional milk, a little nutmeg and salt and pepper and then return the pan to the heat. Cook gently, stirring well, for about 2 minutes until the sauce is smooth and thickened. Serve.

50 g (2 oz) butter
40 g (1½ oz) plain flour
300 ml (½ pint) milk
300 ml (½ pint) single cream or use 600 ml (1 pint) milk in total and omit the cream
freshly grated nutmeg, to taste
salt and pepper

Makes **600 ml (1 pint)**
Prep time **5 minutes**
Cooking time **10 minute**

PARSLEY SAUCE

THIS IS GREAT SERVED WITH FISH OR GAMMON STEAKS.

1 Discard any tough stalks from the parsley and put it into a blender or food processor or blender with half of the stock. Blend until the parsley is very finely chopped.

2 Melt the butter over a medium heat in a heavy-based saucepan until bubbling. Tip in the flour and stir quickly to combine. Cook the mixture gently, stirring constantly with a wooden spoon, for 2 minutes.

3 Remove the pan from the heat and gradually whisk in the parsley-flavoured stock, then the remaining stock, until smooth. Whisk in the milk. Return to the heat and bring to the boil, stirring. Season with salt and pepper. Reduce the heat and continue to cook the sauce for about 5 minutes, stirring frequently, until it is smooth and glossy. The sauce should thinly coat the back of the spoon.

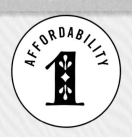

15 g (½ oz) parsley (choose really fresh, fragrant parsley)
250 ml (8 fl oz) Vegetable Stock (see page 244), fish stock or ham stock
25 g (1 oz) butter
25 g (1 oz) plain flour
250 ml (8 fl oz) milk
3 tablespoons single cream
salt and pepper

Makes **600 ml (1 pint)**
Prep time **10 minutes**
Cooking time **10 minute**

RED FRUIT COULIS

TWO OR THREE SUMMER FRUITS, BLENDED AND STRAINED TO PRODUCE A SMOOTH AND COLOURFUL PURÉE, MAKES A USEFUL SAUCE FOR SETTING OFF ALL SORTS OF DESSERTS. USE THE COULIS TO FLOOD THE SERVING PLATES OR DRIZZLE IT AROUND THE EDGES. EITHER WAY, IT WILL REALLY ENHANCE THE PRESENTATION. THIS COULIS IS GREAT SERVED WITH CHOCOLATE CHEESECAKE, VANILLA ICE CREAM, PANCAKES AND FRUIT TARTS OR SIMPLY DRIZZLED OVER GREEK YOGURT.

1 Put the sugar into a small jug and make it up to 50 ml (2 fl oz) with boiling water. Stir until the sugar dissolves and then leave to cool.

2 Remove the redcurrants, if using, from their stalks by running them through the tines of a fork. Place all the fruits in a blender or food processor and blend to a smooth purée, scraping the mixture down from the sides of the bowl if necessary. Blend in the sugar syrup.

3 Pour the sauce into a sieve set over a bowl. Press the purée with the back of a large metal spoon to squeeze out all the juice.

4 Stir in enough lemon juice to make the sauce slightly tangy, then transfer it to a jug. To serve, pour a little coulis on to each serving plate and gently tilt the plate so it is covered in an even layer. Alternatively, use a tablespoon to drizzle the sauce in a ribbon around the edges.

3 tablespoons caster sugar
about 50 ml (2 fl oz) boiling water
500 g (1 lb) fresh ripe summer fruits, such as strawberries, raspberries and redcurrants
2-3 teaspoons lemon juice

Serves **6-8**
Prep time **10 minutes, plus cooling**

VARIATION

Replace up to 200 g (7 oz) of the red fruits with fresh blackcurrants, blackberries or mulberries and add 2-3 tablespoons crème de cassis or an orange liqueur. To make a more autumnal coulis, which is delicious with apple and banana desserts, use only blackberries and double the sugar.

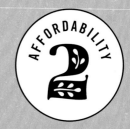

INDEX

ACKNOWLEDGEMENTS

Picture Credits
Dreamstime.com Absente 172 right; Al1962 243 below left; Artofphoto 136 above; Dušan Zidar 243 below right; Mallivan 75 above; Nataliya Arzamasova 173; Pojoslaw 227 left; Sanse293 75 below; Ukrphoto 172 left; Voyagerix 7; Wavebreakmedia Ltd 227 right; Zigzagmtart 243 above right. **istockphoto.com** damircudic 226; FangXiaNuo 136 below; joannawnuk 242; laflor 137 above; Leonardo Patrizi 137 below; monkeybusinessimages 205 right. **Octopus Publishing Group** Craig Robertson 26; David Munns 216 left, 229, 237; Emma Neish 35, 223; Gareth Sambidge 14, 15; Ian Wallace 37, 84, 113, 143, 203; Jason Lowe 133; Lis Parsons 2, 10, 18, 19, 27, 28, 31, 32, 39, 62, 73, 85, 86, 90, 94, 97, 98, 102, 104, 107, 108, 111, 121 below right, 122, 127, 146 below right, 146 above, 159, 165, 167, 169, 175, 179, 186 above right, 189, 209, 216 right, 217 left, 217 right, 218, 220, 221, 222, 232, 233, 235, 236; Sean Myers 191; Stephen Conroy 3 left, 33, 58, 59, 60, 61, 65, 69, 75 centre, 83, 100, 101, 106, 121 below left, 123, 130, 135, 139, 141, 166, 168, 186 above left, 190, 193, 206, 214, 248; Will Heap 3 right, 9, 17, 47, 49, 57, 72, 78, 79, 81, 89, 110, 146 below left, 151, 152, 153, 154, 157, 176, 178, 180, 186 below left, 195, 215, 234; William Lingwood 155, 163; William Reavell 8 left, 34, 40, 41, 43, 76, 121 above right, 132, 147, 181, 192, 194; William Shaw 8 right, 12, 20, 25, 29, 52, 54, 55, 63, 87, 93, 109, 121 above left, 134, 145, 161, 186 below right, 188, 199, 200, 205 left, 213, 224, 239, 240. **Shutterstock** AS Food studio 243 above left; cluckva 20 background; Curioso 4; designelements 60 background; Gencho Petkov 24-25; photastic 12-13; The_Pixel 10-11; vetkit 2-3. **Thinkstock** Hemera Technologies 29 background; Milos Luzanin 35 background.

Publisher Sarah Ford
Editor Pollyanna Poulter
Designers Eoghan O'Brien and Jaz Bahra
Picture Library Manager Jennifer Veall
Assistant Production Controller Meskerem Berhane

Extra recipes by Joanna Farrow
Features writer Cara Frost-Sharratt